READ THIS

Before Changing Your Diet

If you have any health conditions or are on medication, you should check with your physician first before starting this diet. Be aware that strict adherence to this diet may require an adjustment in blood sugar and blood pressure medication with the help of your physician in as little as one day. Despite the description of the improvement of health of the many people described in this book and the positive impact this diet may have on various health conditions, the "Peace Diet" is not intended as treatment for any specific disease.

Dr.Shintani's

Peace Diet™

Cookbook

**The companion book to the
Peace Diet™
on how to lose weight and live longer by
eating for peace of body, mind, and spirit.**

Health Foundation Press

Peace Diet™ Cookbook
© 2016 Terry Shintani, M.D., J.D., M.P.H.

For information contact:
Health Foundation Press
50 S. Beretania St. C-119B
Honolulu, HI 96813

ISBN 9781539001263

Originally Published in the United States of America
The Peace™ Diet Cookbook, Terry Shintani, M.D., J.D., M.P.H.
10 9 8 7 6 5 4 3 2 1

Layout: Lanilane Ocbina
Cover: Gershom Callada

By author of Hawaii's #1 bestseller, *the HawaiiDiet*

Dr. Shintani's
The
Peace Diet™
Cookbook

**The companion book to the Peace Diet™
on how to Lose weight and live longer by eating
for peace of body, mind and spirit**

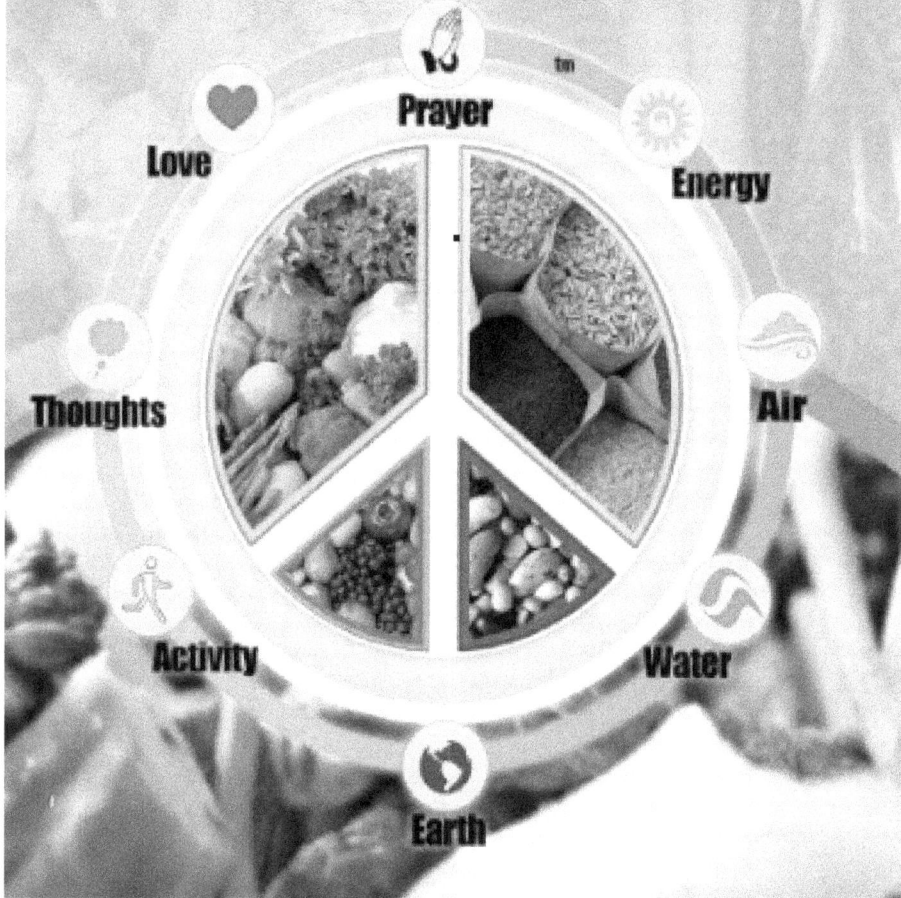

Prayer

Love

Energy

Thoughts

Air

Activity

Water

Earth

Contents

DEDICATION vii
ACKNOWLEDGEMENTS ix
FOREWORD xv
PREFACE xvii
INTRODUCTION...1
RECIPES..11
  WHOLE GRAIN...14
    Easy Cooking, Lots of Uses 15
    Cooking Chart for Grains..15
    Rice Dishes...16
    Ah, Technology! 17
    Gourmet Rice Is a Breeze 17
    Kitchari - An Ayurvedic Weight-Loss and Detox Dish...17
    Simple Kitchari 18
    Effortless Options..19
    Wheat Berry Rice 20
    Stovetop Rice Pilaf..21
    Baked Wild Rice Pilaf 22
    Stovetop Spanish Rice..23
    American Lentil Rice Pilaf..24
    Mung Bean Surprise...25
    Azuki Rice (Sekihan) 26
    Popular, Versatile Pilafs...27
    Healthy Breakfast Alternative 28
    Toasty Cooked Breakfast Cereal................................28
    Quinoa Fruit breakfast...29
    Another Versatile Crowd Pleaser 30
    Steamed Sweet Potatoes or Yams 31
    Orange-Date Glaze 31
  Pasta 32
    Whole Grain Pastas 32

Tomato Vermicelli 34
Vegetarian Ravioli 35
Marinara Sauce...36
Pasta With Eggplant Sauce 37
Pasta with Roasted Vegetables......................................38
Asian Cold Pasta 41
Basic Buckwheat Noodles...43
Asian Dipping Sauce...44
Buckwheat Noodle Medley 45
Asian Pasta Salad 46
VEGETABLES 48
Less Oil, Better Nutrition..49
Salads and Dressings..50
Mark Ellman's Tomato Miso Vinaigrette.......................51
Chinese Lettuce Wraps 52
Thousand Island Dressing 54
Great Caesar Salad 55
Great Caesar Salad Dressing 56
Miso Potato Salad 57
Peter Merriman's Mixed Green Vegetable Salad with Ka'u
Gold® Potatoes 58
Carrot-Celery-Pepper Sticks & Garden Dip 59
Lomi Tomato...60
Fragrant Salad 61
Summer Relish Salad 62
Green Bean Salad..63
Asparagus Artichoke Salad 64
Green Papaya Salad...65
Fresh Citrus Salad 66
Soups..67
Peking Hot & Sour Soup...69
Potato and Corn Chowder 70
Corn Soup...72
Wakame Soup 74
Wakame Onion Mushroom Soup...................................75
Wheat Berry Vegetable Soup...76

Mushroom-Broccoli Noodle Soup 77
Breakfast Miso Soup 78
Cream of Broccoli Soup 79
Portuguese Bean Soup..80
Vegetable Barley Soup 81
Vegetable Entrees...82
Vegetable Stir Fry 82
Mu Shu Vegetables 83
Vegetable Wraps and Mu Shu Vegetable 84
Plum Sauce (Hoi Sin Sauce) 85
Hawaiian Savory Stew 86
Curry Stew 87
Mushroom Vegetable Stew 88
Cajun Jambalaya 89
Spicy Tofu With Cabbage 90
Confetti Rice Stir-Fry...91
Nishime (a form of Japanese stew) 92
Monk's Food...94
Zucchini Caliente 96
Vegetable Side Dishes...97
Vegetable Kebobs 99
Simple Vegetable Kebob..99
Sauces and Gravies 100
Sauces For Steamed Vegetables..............................101
Dijon Mustard Sauce 102
Asian Sauce 102
Oriental Ginger Sauce 103
Miso-Based Sauce 103
Ginger Miso Sauce 104
Curry Sauce 105
Barbecue Sauce 106
Tofu Sauce 108
Tofu Dip Sauce 109
Mediterranean Herb Sauce 110
Steamed Garlic Broccoli 111
Melt-In-Your-Mouth Kabocha Squash 112

Butternut Squash with Whole Wheat, Wild Rice, and Onion
Stuffing..113
Broccoli With Mustard Sauce 115
Baked Eggplant Marinara 116
Wakame with Mixed Vegetables 117
Mock Crabmeat Sauce Over Broccoli...............................118
Broccoli With Mustard Sauce 119
High Calcium Vegetables 120
Zesty Broccoli 122
Sea Vegetables 123
Watercress Sesame Salad...124
Spicy Broccoli...125
Wakame with Carrots..127
Wakame Namasu 128
Ginger Mustard Cabbage with Konbu 129
Vegetable Staples 130
Roasted Potatoes 130
Teriyaki Potatoes...131
Chestnut Stuffing 132
Steamed Sweet Potatoes or Yams 133
BEANS...136
Chunky Three-Bean Chili 138
Barbecue Baked Bean 139
Quick Chili...140
Sweet and Sour Tofu..141
Chickenless Long Rice...142
Srambled Tofu..143
Tofu Nuggets..144
Broiled Falafel..145
Hawaiian Savory Stew 146
Red Chili Lentil Stew...148
Vegetable Stew..150
Vegetable Laulau 151
Maui Tacos Black Bean Burrito...152
Dick Allgire's Lazy Enchiladas 153
Ann's Garbanzo Casserole 155

Beans and Carrot Stew 156
Zip Burritos 157
Pronto Bean and Rice Burritos...............................158
Chapati Burritos 159
Fresh Salsa Caliente 160
Mock Tuna 161
Bean Dips 162
EMWL Bean Dip 162
Black Bean Dip 164
Simple Hummus..165
FRUITS 168
Apple-Strawberry Jel 169
Baked Apple With Raisin Sauce 171
Peach Crisp...172
Quick Apple Pie 173
Iced Fruit Cream 174
A Few More Sweet Delights....................................175
Strawberry-Banana Pudding 175
Honey Almond Fruit Cocktail.................................176
GLYCEMIC INDEX (GI) AND
DR. SHINTANI'S
FOOD MASS INDEX (SMI) TABLES.........................177

DEDICATION

To the Almighty Father, the Great Physician, His Son, the Prince
of Peace, and all the messengers of peace He has sent to this
Earth including YOU.

ACKNOWLEDGEMENTS

There are so many people to thank in producing this book as it has taken a lifetime of my medical training and practice to have the background to write it. I first want to say thanks to my recently departed mentor, Kenneth Francis Brown, with whom I shared a vision of health and peace. He helped me start the non-profit foundation, the Hawaii Health Foundation, where all royalties from this book will go. I want to thank my board members who have supported our work for years including Dr. Earl Bakken, inventor of the wearable pacemaker and founder of Medtronic, (the largest medical device company in the world), Hooipo DeCambra, a Robert Wood Johnson Leadership awardee, Jim Jacoby, one of the nation's leading environmentally-conscious land developer. My hanai mother, Dr. Agnes Cope, my hanai brother, Kamaki Kanahele, Al Harrington (of Hawaii 5-0 fame) and my attorney and law school classmate and friend, Ronald Sakamoto.

I also want to thank Dr. T. Colin Campbell, principal investigator of the China Diet Study, one of the greatest nutrition researchers, who is another mentor of mine. His work has developed much of the science that supports the healthfulness of a plant-based diet. Thanks also goes to Michio Kushi, the founder of the American Macrobiotic movement, who taught me the connection between diet and spirit when I first met him in the 1970's. I also want to acknowledge my friend, Keith Tamura, who introduced me to Macrobiotics when he turned his asthma around with a change in diet.

Thanks also goes to Dr. John McDougall, a true pioneer in plant-based diets for the reversal of disease, who turned his Hawaii practice over to me when he left for California. He was putting science to this concept in the '70's – long before some of the currently well-known proponents of a plant-based diet. I also owe a debt of gratitude to Dr. Walter Willett, my nutrition professor at Harvard University who is now Chief of Nutrition, and along with Dr. Campbell, is one of the greatest nutrition researchers in the world. I also want to acknowledge another one of my Harvard professors, Dr. William Castelli, principal investigator of the Framingham Study, arguably the greatest study on nutrition and heart disease. I am ever grateful for Dr. Claire Hughes, the first Native Hawaiian registered dietitian and co-author of some of my early writings, Dr. Kekuni Blaisdell, my teacher and professor of medicine, and Helen Kanawaliwali O'Connor, a Native Hawaiian healer who was always my partner on our Hawaiian Health projects. Thanks also goes to Dr. Rosanne Harrigan, Chair of the Department of Complementary and Alternative Medicine, who keeps our important work at the University of Hawaii Medical School of Medicine moving forward.

I also have the highest regard for Dr. Keith Block, author of "Life Over Cancer" and founder of the Block Center for Integrative Cancer Therapy; and also Dr. Michael Gregor, whose website www.nutritionfacts.org is the best nutrition science website on the planet. I consulted them both on a number of nutrition and health issues.

My spiritual teachers have been equally important in the development of this book. While I am Christian and the Prior of the Priory of Hawaii of the Knights of the Orthodox Order of St. John Russian Grand Priory, I owe much gratitude to my parents, Robert and Emi, who taught me both Christian and Buddhist values. I also must thank my adoptive Hawaiian mother, Dr. Agnes Cope, the Chair of the Elders Council of the traditional Hawaiian healers, and my adoptive brother, Kahu Kamaki

Kanahele, Director of the Native Hawaiian Healing Center, who taught me principles of Hawaiian spiritual healing. He has done prayers with the Dalai Lama and Mother Theresa while working in Washington D.C.

I must also acknowledge the profound influence of the late Dr. Mits Aoki (nicknamed "the Cosmic Dancer") on my understanding of life, death and spirit. He was my Religion professor and often taught in my spiritual development programs. I am also grateful to Countess Nicholas Bobrinskoy, the Grande Dame and Chancellor of the Knights of the Orthodox Order of St. John Russian Grand Priory, who is the great proponent of the continuation of the nearly 1000-year tradition of service of the Hospitallers of St. John, and also Dame Commander, Dr. Sandra Rose Michael, who initiated the creation of Prior of Hawaii and who is the creator of the EES scalar energy generator. I must also acknowledge QiGong GrandMaster, Dr. Effie Chow, for her wisdom that has helped me to understand much about energy medicine.

I also want to acknowledge the spiritual influence and universal teachings of Dr. Jerry Jampolsky, and Dr. Diane Cirincione-Jampolsky, founders of Attitudinal Healing and the use of the 12 Principles of Attitudinal Healing in this book. Thanks also goes to Dr. Diane Nomura, Administrator of the Hawaii Health Foundation and the long time co-host of our radio show, "Healing And You" (which can be heard on AM 1080 in Honolulu or on http://www.kwai1080am.com/ on Sundays at 8pm HST) for many years of helping me keep the Hawaii Health Foundation and our programs on track and for always insisting on including prayer in our programs. She is the author of the book "What The Health" (www.Lulu.com). I would also like to thank Pastor Jeffrey Yamashita, my baptismal pastor for his spiritual support.

Special appreciation goes to Dr. Patricia Bragg, a true "health crusader" who carries on the legacy of the legendary Dr. Paul Bragg, through the Bragg Live Food Products company, and the Director of the company, Dr. John Westerdahl, who have been inspirations in the field of health. They have been consistent sponsors of my radio show along with Down To Earth health food stores who has generously helped my Foundation to put on my "Reverse Disease in 10 Days" Programs. I also want to express my appreciation for my chefs who cooked for my 10 Day health Programs. I consider them my "kitchen pharmacists" including Leslie Ashburn, OriAnn Li, Kathy Maddux, Alyssa Moreau, and Steve Nochese.

I also need to express my appreciation for the Mokichi Okada Association who allows me to use space at their beautiful Wellness Center in Hawaii to house the clinic of the Department of Complementary and Alternative Medicine of the University of Hawaii Medical School. I also appreciate Dr. Raj Kumar, clinical psychologist and meditation teacher and the Gandhi International Institute of Peace for trusting me to be the Chair of their Advisory Board. I don't have permission or space to name the many generous volunteers individually who have blessed our project with their time and effort. They have helped with so many aspects of our work from photography, to cooking, serving food, assisting with set-up, Internet activities and much more, that make our Foundation viable with the modest funds that we have.

I want to thank Pastora Lanilane Ocbina for doing the layout and her associate Gershom Callada, who put together the beautiful graphics in this book. I also want to thank the editor of my book, Dr. Diane Chesson, who is a consummate professional in her work.

Thanks also goes to my family, my brother, Arthur, his wife, Yuko who run our Integrative Wellness Center. Special thanks my wife, Stephanie, and my children, Tracie and Nickie who have put up with me, helped me, and been the source of my strength over the years. Most of all, I thank the Lord for all of these people and the blessings I have been so fortunate to enjoy in my life and for the underlying truths found in this book.

FOREWORD

by Dr. T. Colin Campbell
Professor Emeritus, Cornell University
and author of the "China Study" and "Whole"

I met Dr. Shintani in the early 1990's at an international conference called "Food Choices 2000". One of the first things I noticed about him was that he was a unique medical doctor who had a degree in nutrition from Harvard University. At that conference, I learned about his work with the traditional Hawaiian diet. He worked with arguably one of the most challenging populations with high rates of obesity, diabetes, cancer, and heart disease. He demonstrated that with a change in diet, these diseases could be reversed.

What I thought was intriguing was that the diet that he recommended was fully in line with what I found in the China Diet Study that I had conducted with my colleagues at Oxford and University of Beijing. He used a diet that was low in animal products, low in processed food, and low in fat. Despite the fact that it was high in carbohydrates, he demonstrated that this kind of diet could induce weight loss and improved control of blood sugar, cholesterol and blood sugar.

Because of his findings and his academic background in medicine and nutrition, I invited him to be a visiting professor for one of my classes at Cornell University. It was important for students to hear about Dr. Shintani's work and his finding that a change in diet could induce health improvement that could rival the benefits of prescription medication.

This book describes a dietary approach that I think is excellent for preventing and even reversing a number of diseases. It is certainly good for weight control as he has demonstrated in his peer-reviewed publications. He also describes an approach to nutrition in dealing with whole foods rather than single nutrients that is consistent with some of the concepts in my more recent book, "Whole".

I find Dr. Shintani's work to be very impressive and certainly founded on excellent scientific principles. He actually takes people who are overweight and takes people who have diabetes for example and he reverses it. He makes people better. The proof is in the pudding.

T. Colin Campbell
Professor Emeritus, Cornell University

PREFACE

This Cookbook is the companion book to the Peace Diet(tm) book on how to lose weight, control chronic disease, and live longer by eating for peace of body, mind and spirit. It contains 102 delicious recipes that are consistent with the principles of the "Peace Diet(tm)". The Preface, Foreword and Introduction in this book come from the "Peace Diet(tm) book to give you an idea what the Peace Diet is about. If you don't already have one, you can obtain a "Peace Diet(tm)" book at www.PeaceDiet.org.

I have been conducting health programs for over 25 years now and consistently get people to lose excess pounds, get healthy enough to get off at least some of their medication, and sometimes find inner peace. I've had the good fortune to be able to combine my nutrition background with my practice as a medical doctor along with principles that I learned from my spiritual teachers.

In the early 1990's the U.S. Secretary of Health and Human Services, Donna Shalala gave my health program a national award. It was for the effectiveness of my whole-person health program that included diet, lifestyle, and spiritual principles in a high health-risk Native Hawaiian community. With the results of the program, I demonstrated that by returning an unhealthy population to a traditional diet and lifestyle, their obesity, diabetes, high blood pressure, and other health ailments could easily be remedied.

I hoped that with the added reputation and notoriety that came with such a prestigious award, I might be able to reach many people with a message of health. I have done some of that, especially in Hawaii and the Native Hawaiian community where they arguably have more health problems than any other

American sub-group as a result of poverty and obesity-related disease. My health books have reached around the world - some of them translated into Spanish, Japanese, and Chinese, and I have been featured in the Encyclopedia Britannica because of the promising results of my program. Ultimately, however, I would like to take it a step further and help people reach their health and spiritual aspirations as well through the practice of the diet and lifestyle described in this book. Through my experience, I have found that the best diet is one that helps you find inner peace - and then weight control and health follow naturally. When people find themselves on a diet that helps them calm their spirit - the way many people of wisdom have done over millennia, - excess pounds melt away and their health returns. After all, if your spirit is not healthy, then your body and mind are not totally healthy either. And if you nurture the total health of your spirit, then body and mind will follow.

You are the reason this book was written. It is my hope that it will inform and inspire you to choose the path to health, success, happiness and peace, and that through you others will be informed and inspired. In doing so, I hope to contribute to the movement promoting world health and world peace, one person, one spirit at a time.

Just about every person can heal with the proper diet based on the "Peace Plate," with the eight practices described in this book – and with the help of the Almighty. When healthy in body, mind and spirit, a person can do great things. And when we work together with a healthy spirit, we can heal the world. As the great Mahatma Gandhi once said, "*Be the change you want to see*".

My Father Had Cancer

Since childhood, I have been aware of the spiritual side of life. I learned to pray when I was very young. When I was 6 months old in 1951, my father was diagnosed with colon cancer. They took out the whole left side of his colon and left him with a permanent colostomy. They said he would be lucky to live another couple of years. My father had a second surgery when I was just 3 years old, and I remember feeling afraid of losing him. Imagine what it's like for a 3-year-old to understand the meaning of the word "metastasis" (the spreading of cancer)? So I began to pray - every night. *"Dear God. Please don't let Dad die of cancer. . ."*

Every single night I prayed that simple prayer - for years - decades. Fortunately, he lived another 40 years and never died of cancer. I will always believe that my prayers had something to do with his survival. After all, how many people do you know of who survived colon cancer in the 1950's? Little did I know then that my Dad having had cancer ultimately, decades later, would lead to my finding a connection between diet, health and peace, and to dedicating my career to helping enhance the lives of as many people as I can.

From Cancer to Peace

Because of this experience, from a young age, I wanted to explore better ways to deal with cancer than what was offered conventionally. After all, doctors didn't seem to have any good answers for my father, and my uncle, who later developed colon cancer and died several months after his diagnosis. I looked into Oriental Medicine, Ayurvedic Medicine, the Gerson Diet, and even Laetrile, purportedly an anticancer substance found in apricot pits.

I first heard about the concept of diet as a path to world peace when I was looking for alternative approaches to dealing with cancer.   When I got into law school, I struggled to keep up because I was tired all the time. A friend of mine suggested I try looking into macrobiotics to improve my health and increase my energy. Macrobiotics is primarily known for its dietary approach to health and cancer.   It is a whole system of diet and lifestyle that is based on balancing the energies of yin and yang.   My friend said that it may help me with my school work. He said that it helped him get rid of his allergies, and his energy and mental alertness improved. Desperate, I tried it. I started eating according to its dietary guidelines.   It worked better than I ever expected. My energy returned, and my mind cleared up.   My mood and my grades improved. I was determined to learn more about it.

As I began to explore macrobiotics, I was intrigued to learn of many reported cases of people who had reversed cancer, heart disease, diabetes and other diseases using macrobiotics. Interestingly, "One peaceful world" is one of their mottos, and there is a book by that title published by my teacher, Michio Kushi. This puzzled me at first because it seemed strange to talk about world peace in the teachings of healing.

My teacher, Michio Kushi, the father of the American Macrobiotic movement was in his youth a brilliant political science scholar who studied world government at Tokyo University and Columbia University. Because he witnessed the horrors of World War II and the deaths of many of his close friends in the fire-bombings of Tokyo, his passion was to create a movement to end the need for war. So he diligently studied world government at two of the best universities in the world.

Everything changed when he met George Ohsawa, the founder of macrobiotics. Ohsawa told Kushi that he was a fool if he thought studying world government could lead ultimately to world peace. If the people are unhealthy in body, mind, and spirit, explained Ohsawa, the government will be corrupt no matter how good the governmental system may be. Conversely, if the people are healthy in body mind and spirit, then the government would be healthy, spiritually guided, and world peace would be possible. Ohsawa encouraged Kushi to promote the macrobiotic diet as the pathway to the health of body, mind, and spirit.

I too made this mission my life's path and, in addition to formal training in nutrition at Harvard University after medical school, I have also been formally trained in macrobiotics and the principles of Oriental Medicine at the Kushi Institute and trained in traditional Hawaiian healing by my adopted native Hawaiian family. Remarkably, if you dig deeply enough, you will find that these divergent approaches arrive at the same fundamental truth. You will find that they all acknowledge that the best approach to health is a holistic approach to health including body, mind and spirit, and that the best diet for health and spiritual development is based on whole, unprocessed plant-based food.

Many Have Connected Diet and Peace
My first exposure to how diet affects one's spirit was in experiencing the food served at Buddhist funerals. I grew up in a mixed Christian and Buddhist family, and I noticed that after Buddhist funerals, they would always serve vegetarian food. It was called "shojin ryori" or spiritual development meals. The Buddhist masters believed that plant-based food nurtured the spirit, and that animal-based food would bind your spirit to the earth and make it difficult to spiritually support the departed spirit. For similar reasons "jai," also called "monks' food" in Chinese Buddhist tradition, is vegetarian.

To my surprise, few mainstream experts – scientists, theologians, philosophers, doctors alike – ever talked about the relationship between food and spiritual development. Yet there it was in the Bible and, when I looked further, in the practices of many religions and cultures. Despite differences in belief and practice between Christians and Buddhists, both religions revered plant-based foods.

In the Bible, Genesis 1:29 states that the original God-given diet was plant-based where it says the food includes *"every plant bearing seed . . . and every tree with seed in its fruit . . . "* for humans to eat. In the book of Daniel, Daniel insisted on eating "vegetables" instead of the "king's meat" and he was found to be healthier and better than the king's other advisors. This appreciation of plant-based food is similar to the Buddhist tradition of "shojin ryori" or "spiritual development food" as described above, and to the vegetarian tradition of the Hindu faith.

Many Religions Equate Plant-Based Diet & Peace
On further investigation, I found many more sources from various religions all over the world and from great philosophers and teachers describing how a plant-based diet positively influences our mental and spiritual development. I never read anything purporting that a meat-centered diet could do the same. Quite the contrary, sources suggest that animal flesh when consumed hinders the peace-loving spirit.

Modern Movement toward Peace & Plant-Based Diet
Some modern authors too describe the same truth about the relationship between diet and spiritual development, and are worthy of notice. Most notably are books by Dr. Gabriel Cousens who wrote *Spiritual Nutrition,*[1] Stephen Rosen who wrote *Food for the Spirit,*[2] Michio Kushi and Alex Jack who wrote <u>One Peaceful World</u> and Will Tuttle who wrote the <u>*World Peace Diet.*</u>[3]

Each of these books describes the healthfulness of a plant-based diet and its value in promoting spiritual development and a sense of personal peace.

My Unique Perspective

But I believe I have a unique perspective as a nutritionist, practicing physician, and medical school professor. I am one of relatively few physicians who have credentials in nutrition, have conducted research, and also practice medicine with real patients. I have also been formally trained in what might be called "alternative" health systems such as macrobiotics and traditional Hawaiian healing, (the ancient healing arts of Hawaii). I have also engaged in spiritual development training that incorporates diet and lifestyle to improve health. I have personally experienced an elevation of spirit while on a strict "Peace Diet" for spiritual development.

When following the guidelines of the Peace Diet, I have personally experienced an elevation in energy, mood, and awareness. I have had experiences and insights of things to happen in the future that I could not explain otherwise except that the Diet elevated my consciousness, enabling me to tap into some higher consciousness. I have accomplished things in my career that I never thought possible. For example, I credit this higher consciousness that opened me to the guidance of the Almighty with how we were able to create a health program that won a National award with essentially no funding. It was so successful that we were featured in Newsweek, CBS This Morning, CNN news, Dateline NBC and in the Encyclopedia Britannica.

In addition, for over 20 years I have conducted health programs based on a plant-based diet and improved the health of thousands of people who have come through my programs and practice. I have seen individuals lose hundreds of pounds and cholesterol numbers, blood pressures, blood sugars, and countless ailments improve on a plant-based diet based on the concepts I recommend in this book. It has always impressed me that a diet that is good for the spirit is also the best diet for the mind and body.

As with my other books, this book is about nutrition, and yet the focus is a little different from my other books. First, it is a much simplified version of the diet that I recommend. It is certainly about improving our health, losing excess pounds, and feeling better than ever. But it is also about a missing element in nutrition that is often neglected but in many ways may be more important than dealing with weight, diabetes, heart disease, and other chronic ailments. It is about how diet affects our personal peace and even world peace as described by many philosophers and writers before me.

This focus on nutrition leading to peace, coupled with my career-long practice of "lifestyle medicine" and "whole-person" health programs where I experienced not just the medical and health results of a good diet but also the spiritual effects, as well as my witnessing greater intuition, more lucid dreams, and near psychic effects has led me to write this book. It is my hope that it may help you in your own path to health, enlightenment and peace.

> *"Behold, I have given you every plant yielding seed which is upon the face of all the earth, and every tree with seed in its fruit; you shall have then for food."*
> *-   Genesis 1:29*

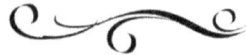

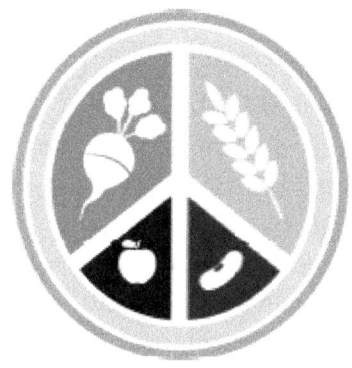

INTRODUCTION

This Cookbook is the companion book to the Peace Diet(tm) book on how to lose weight, control chronic disease, and live longer by eating for peace of body, mind and spirit. It contains 102 delicious recipes that are consistent with the principles of the "Peace Diet(tm)". The Preface, Foreword and Introduction in this book come from the "Peace Diet(tm) book to give you an idea what the Peace Diet is about. If you don't already have one, you can obtain a "Peace Diet(tm)" book at www.PeaceDiet.org.

The Book You've Been Looking For

This may be the book you have been looking for. The fact that you are reading these words in this book is no accident. Call it synchronicity, coincidence, guidance from the universe or the hand of God; in whatever way you choose to describe it, you are reading this book for a reason that may change your life.

You have been guided to these pages to explore this way of controlling your weight, optimizing your health, reducing your need for medication, and elevating your mood and spirit. In this book I want to share a simple secret of the ages with you. I want to show you how to control your weight, reverse disease, chronic pain, and the aging process by creating peace of body, peace of mind, and peace of spirit.

The Best Diet in the World

I want to introduce you to the best diet in the world. This is not just my opinion. It is the opinion of many people in the field of health, doctors, nutritionists, celebrities, athletes, leaders, and especially great souls throughout history. The principles behind this diet are found in modern health books, ancient holy books, popular books, and scientific journals. This diet allows you to eat as much as you want and still lose weight, while at the same time regaining your health. Many people on this diet have regained energy and reduced or eliminated their need for medication. Here is what one patient says:

"I've lost weight - about 50 pounds." . . . I was taking 75 units [of insulin] a day and taking four high blood pressure pills. . . But after 10 days, my insulin count went down to 5 units a day and my cholesterol went down to about 100 and I don't need blood pressure medicine anymore." Ronald N.

This diet, which I call the Peace Diet, has allowed some people to lose over a hundred pounds without counting a single calorie. Many have seen their aches and pains disappear, their headaches gone, and their fatigue and depression evaporate. Other people swear that it has improved their energy and spiritual development.

"Somehow, eating this way, my mind is clearer, my consciousness is elevated and my prayers seem more effective." John W.

Why do I call it the best diet in the world? Well, what other diet allows you to lose weight without counting calories or portion size, has been shown to reverse heart disease, diabetes,

2

hypertension and other health problems, is associated with better mood, and has been recommended through the ages for spiritual development? In addition, it helps the environment, reduces the suffering of animals, and reduces karmic debt. It's a diet that produces real results in real people who see their blood sugar, cholesterol, blood pressure, and many other ailments improve. It's a diet that helps people feel better physically, mentally, emotionally, and spiritually.

Not a Fad Diet

The Peace Diet is not a "fad diet." It is not a diet that carries the name of a famous doctor. It does not bear the name of some trendy place or food. It is not named after some catchy principle that has been invented in the last few years. It is not based on one or two nutrients or metabolic process. Instead, it is based on principles that are thousands of years old and validated by modern science. It is based on a few timeless principles that bring into play the full complexity of the interaction of whole food on the whole of human physiology.

The Peace Diet developed out of my own search for health and energy in which I discovered a way of eating that ultimately changed my life. Changes to my eating habits not only caused natural weight loss and improvement in health, but also elevated my mind and my spirit. This has enabled me to find the mental energy to earn four college degrees, and the spiritual guidance to apply this knowledge to help those who need it most. In a nutshell, this is what I have learned since adhering to the Peace Diet in my own life:

"Sow a healthy diet, reap a healthy body; sow a healthy body, reap a healthy spirit; sow a healthy spirit, reap a healthy world."

It is my deep belief that a truly healthy world means a peaceful world, and that peace within a person leads to peace in his/her interactions with others.

Diet for Body, Mind, and Spirit

I have learned that a diet that is healthy for the spirit is going to be the best diet for the mind and body. Think about it. Ask yourself, if your spirit is not healthy, are you ever truly and completely healthy? Ask yourself, if you are taking medication, are you every truly healthy? Is your body ever at peace? Or do the medications fix one problem and cause problems elsewhere? Then ask yourself, what is the best diet and lifestyle that supports the health of your body, mind and spirit?

If you want to know the answer, consider the wisdom of spiritually developed people throughout the ages and couple it to modern science and actual clinical results of people who have tried it. Then, consider trying the Peace Diet because it is a way of life to support the health of your spirit as well and your mind and body. And because it will support the health of spirit, mind and body, it is also the best way to lose weight, get physically healthy, reduce or eliminate the need for medication, and keep you truly healthy in the long run.

Why the Peace Diet?

I call it the Peace Diet because I have found that eating in a way that brings peace and harmony to your bodily processes brings natural weight control, and optimal physical, mental and spiritual health. In other words, I have found that eating in a way that minimizes the metabolic wars going on in your body brings natural weight control and reversal of disease, as well as the elevation of your mind and spirit. My experience and that of others is that if you follow the Peace Diet carefully, you may find yourself feeling less stress, less discomfort, and more energy,

4

calmness, and personal peace as a result.

In the process of gaining peace of body, mind and spirit, you may find pounds falling off and your health returning. It does so because no longer will your body have to fight so many metabolic battles that result in fatigue, overweight and disease. No longer will you have to battle your hunger drive to control your weight. Your body will function the way nature intended it to function. People throughout the ages have used this diet to help them find inner peace. People in modern times can use it to find weight control and health as well.

I also call this the "Peace Diet" because it is based on a diagram that looks like the simple universal "Peace Sign" that describes the diet in a simple, easy-to-use manner as you will see. The fact that people find natural weight loss and improvement in their blood pressure, blood sugar, and cholesterol is probably the best evidence that it is the right kind of diet to follow.

The Peace Diet for Weight Control
The Peace Diet is a proven method for effective weight control. I spent 18 years at a community health center in Hawaii serving an ethnically mixed, largely native Hawaiian population, one of the most obesity-prone populations in the world. I worked in family practice and preventive medicine programs. Some of my patients were 300, 400, 500, even 600 pounds; my largest was 890 pounds. Many were living in poverty, which meant that they tended to eat more convenience food and fast food. Of course, whether we live in poverty or not, processed, convenience-type food greatly increases our risk of obesity.

Perhaps the most obvious and immediate benefit of the Peace Diet, which calls for removing processed foods from one's diet, is weight loss. Margaret, one of my most memorable patients, lost 70 pounds in 6 months. She wound up losing nearly half of her 243 pounds-- and has kept it off for years. This is what Margaret says about being on my health Program:

"When I started the program, I weighed 243 pounds. Currently, I weigh about 128 pounds. I'm kinda going in between 125 and 130 pounds. The other thing too is that I thought, now my outside matches my inside. You know, now I look like how I feel on the inside. My cholesterol used to be 223. Now, almost two years after the program, it stays at around 131. I recommend this program to anyone, and if you don't make it complicated, if you follow it, it's really not hard." Margaret F.

The Peace Diet and Health
As you can see from this participant's example, it isn't just weight that is controlled. Cholesterol is reduced, sometimes as much as 100 points in three weeks. Blood pressure improves, sometimes in as little as one or two days. Blood sugar levels are also positively affected by the Peace Diet, despite the fact that there is no portion-size restriction and it is typically high in carbohydrates.

Another of my patients, who was on 120 units of insulin before she began to follow the Peace Diet, was able to control her blood sugar without taking insulin shots within only ten days. In her words:

When I started the program, I was taking 120 units of insulin, and on the 10th day, I had to stop taking insulin altogether because my blood sugars were getting too low. Now, one year later, I've lost around 35 to 40 pounds and I'm still off insulin. Joanne G

The Peace Diet and Spirit
People following this eating program notice that their energy

increases and their mood is better. Here is the comment of another Peace Diet follower:

What I found is that with this program, I feel very light, I have a lot of energy. Arlene R.

I feel wonderful. Every day I get up, and I feel happy. Melissa T.

In addition, some people start noticing inexplicably that their spiritual consciousness increases. This is just what is described in ancient texts and quotes from spiritual teachers. I'll continue to point out again and again that the best diet for health is one that improves the spirit as well as the body and mind.

"When one becomes a vegetarian, it purifies the soul" – Isaac Bashevis Singer, Author, Nobel laureate

"A vegetarian diet elevates the spirit and makes meditation much more effective" Sooriya Kumar, www.mounafarm.org

The Peace Plate
The Peace Plate is how I describe the way the general proportions of food should look on your plate. To picture this, think of the way the peace sign itself looks: a circle divided down the center vertically with dividing lines starting at the center of the vertical line and angling downwards symmetrically on each side, ending at the edge of the circle. Now imagine that there is a peace sign on your dinner plate.

Dr. Shintani's
PEACE PLATE

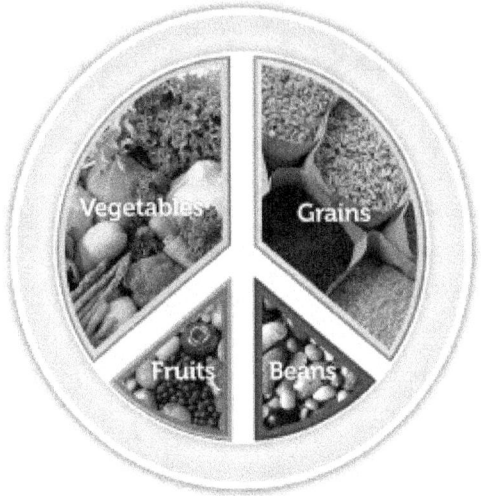

On the left side of the plate, the larger top section covering about 30 to 35% of the plate should be filled with vegetables, with the smaller section at the bottom left reserved for fruit-- about 15% to 20% of the plate. On the right hand side, whole grains should occupy the larger top section, again representing about 30 to 35% of the plate. Beans & legumes round out the lower right space of the Peace Plate configuration, occupying the remaining 15-20% of the circle.

If you follow the guidelines described in this book for constructing the Peace Plate at every meal, a process which also includes using unprocessed food, chewing properly, eating with gratitude, eating foods in season, and eating in harmony with your locality, you will have a diet that supports good health.

Your diet will also be a rough modern equivalent to the *"shojin ryori,"* or the Zen concept of diet for spiritual development, which is discussed later in this book.

Whole Person Peace Plan Includes 8 Enhancing Factors

This diet doesn't stop with the dinner plate, however. Supporting the Peace Plate are eight enhancements forming the basis of a lifestyle that can improve health and elevate the spirit. The first four are environmental: energy, air, water, and earth. In other words, it is important to optimize your exposure to energy, clean air, pure water, and natural elements of the earth, by which I mean minerals and molecules.

The second four enhancements to the Peace Plate are based on intention: activity, thoughts, love, and prayer. As you read through this book and come to understand all the guidelines of the Peace Diet, from the food you eat to the environment you surround yourself with, to the behavior you employ, you will see that all of it is consistent with the recommendations of both ancient wisdom and modern science.

The Peace Diet is Based on Timeless Principles

The Peace Diet is based on timeless principles that have been taught for millennia by physicians and philosophers alike. Some of the principles may be found in Ayurvedic medicine as well as traditional Chinese medicine. It may be found in Buddhist philosophy as well as the Holy Bible. The effectiveness of these principles of the Peace Diet has also been supported by modern peer-reviewed science. The ancient principles combined with modern science will help you to see that when you have peace at the molecular level you will lay the foundation for the peace and health of body, mind, and spirit.

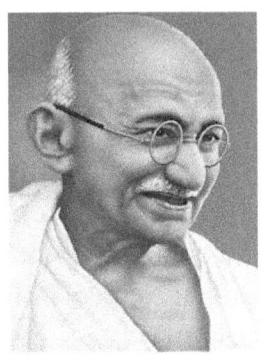

"The greatness of a nation and its moral progress can be judged by the way its animals are treated."

"To my mind, the life of a lamb is no less precious than that of a human being."

Mahatma Gandhi, statesman and philosopher (1869-1948)

RECIPES

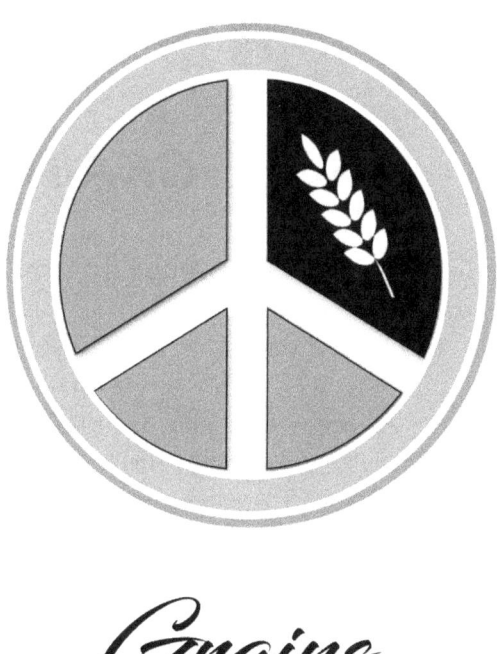

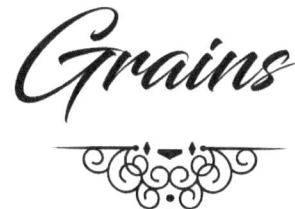

Grains

WHOLE GRAIN

Grains have been a major food source in many areas of the world throughout history, and for good reason. They're loaded with protein, fiber, vitamins, and minerals. They are inexpensive to buy and easy to cook with. You can use them in soups, salads, side dishes, and main dishes. They are delicious in everything from breakfast cereals 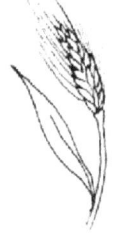 to pasta, to bread and even in desserts. The key is to be sure that you're using whole grains, not refined grains. Refined grains such as those found in white flour and white rice cause grains to be stripped of fiber and nutrients, but using whole grains is beneficial even to the point of reducing the risk of diabetes, heart disease, stroke, and cancer.

Whole grains provide both soluble and insoluble fiber. Soluble fiber lowers blood cholesterol, while insoluble fiber prevents constipation and can help protect against certain cancers. Whole grains are also beneficial by creating a feeling of fullness, which can help dieters to eat less.

There are hundreds of different grains. In the list below I've chosen common varieties that you will easily find in your

14

supermarket or health food store. Remember to store all grains in a cool, dry place to retain longest shelf life (which can be months).

Easy Cooking, Lots of Uses

Often people avoid cooking with whole grains because they're not sure how to prepare them, but the chart below demonstrates that it's fairly easy. Always try to keep grains as close to their natural state as possible. Here are some fast, easy recipes to get you started.

Cooking Chart for Grains

1 cup of grain	Regular Pot		Pressure cooker	
	cups of water	time	cups of water	time
Rolled oats	2-2.5*	20-25 min.	n/a	n/a
Brown Rice	2	40-55 min.	1.5-1.75	30-40 min.
Buckwheat	2-2.5*	2-2.5 hrs.	n/a	n/a
Pearled Barley	2	25-30min.	1.25	15 min.
Hulled Barley	2.5-3*	1.5-1.75 hrs.	2.5	20-25 min.
Bulgur Wheat	1.5-2*	20 min.	n/a	n/a
Whole Wheat	2	1.5-2 hrs.	1.5	20-25 min.
Oats, Rye	2	1-2 hrs.	1.5	20-25 min.
Millet	2	25-35 min.	1.5	15 min.

*Lower number will yield a slightly chewier grain.
Higher number will yield a slightly softer grain.

Rice Dishes

More people eat rice worldwide than any other single food. Rice is rich in beneficial complex carbohydrates, low in fat and calories, and rich in nutrients when it has not been refined. Rice aids digestion and has been found to assist in lowering the risk for diabetes, obesity, high cholesterol, and heart disease.

Brown rice is the most nutritious form of rice and the only one that contains vitamin E. This is because only the inedible husk has been removed. It is full of satisfying complex carbohydrates, fiber, B complex vitamins, and other nutrients. It has a nutty flavor and chewy texture; it takes slightly longer to cook than white rice. Brown rice comes in many varieties: long grain, short grain, and medium grain. You can choose from basmati rice, jasmine rice, arborio, plain brown, Thai black, long grain wild rice, and risotto. Here are some characteristics of just a few of the varieties:

- Basmati rice is very fragrant, comes from India and Pakistan, and doubles in length when it's cooked. It can be substituted for regular rice in most recipes.
- Arborio rice is a creamy white rice grown in Italy and often used for classic Italian risotto dishes. It can also be used in paella and rice pudding.
- Jasmine rice was originally from Thailand but is now grown in the United States. It is similar to basmati and good in Southeast Asian dishes.

For delicious, easy-to-prepare dishes, experiment with some of these varieties to find out which ones appeal most to you. But remember to choose brown rice or the darker varieties since they have the most nutrition.

Ah, Technology!

Cooking rice and other grains has become easier -- basically foolproof! Automatic rice cookers are a great aid because they turn themselves off automatically when the rice is cooked. All you have to do is put in the proper amount of water. These cookers do a good job of steaming rice as well. Foolproof directions are included with the appliance.

Gourmet Rice Is a Breeze

What's better than eating "gourmet" food that's been easy, breezy to prepare? Not much! That's what you can have when you prepare basmati brown rice. Basmati is known as the "King of Rice." Originating in India, it's been enjoyed by their elite for centuries. It's rich and aromatic and is enjoyed by almost everyone who tries it (it's my personal favorite). Easy to find and easy to prepare, cook it like any other brown rice.

Kitchari - An Ayurvedic Weight-Loss and Detox Dish

A simple variation on Basmati rice makes it into "kitchari" which is a popular ayurvedic health dish. Some people will eat just kitchari for several days to do a dietary cleanse or detox. "Kitchari" simply means "mixture". For this dish, it is mainly a mixture of Basmati rice with mung beans and some spices. Here is a simple recipe and also a list of ingredients to make it more elaborate.

Simple Kitchari

1 cup	basmati rice
1 cup	yellow split mung dal
1/2 tsp	turmeric
1 small	handful cilantro leaves, chopped
6 cups	water
	Sea salt and pepper to taste.

Wash the rice and mung dal twice, using plenty of water. If you have time, let the mung dal soak for a few hours before cooking, to help with digestibility.

Add rice, dal, turmeric and cilantro to the water. Bring to a boil, and boil 5 minutes uncovered, stirring occasionally.

Turn down heat to low, and cover, leaving the lid slightly ajar. Cook until tender, about 25 to 30 minutes. Season with salt and pepper to taste.

Here are additional optional seasonings to add with the turmeric if you have time and the ingredients.

1/4 teaspoon	mustard seeds
1 1/2 teaspoons	cumin
1 teaspoon	fenugreek
1. tsp	fennel
1 tsp	coriander powder
1 tsp	fresh ginger
1 pinch	Hing (acefetida)

Effortless Options

Another good thing about whole grains is their flexibility. You can vary the overall taste effortlessly by adding other types of grains to your brown rice. Then add in some vegetables and top off with some sauces or gravies. All your choices can be both nutritious and delicious. The variations are endless, depending on your imagination and taste.

Here are two suggestions, just to get you started:

- Add in some wild rice. This rice came from the seed of a swamp grass and in the past grew only in the wild, but now it is also cultivated. It has an interesting woodsy flavor and is packed with iron, protein, niacin and fiber.
- How about wheat berries? Wheat berries are whole, unprocessed kernels of wheat, so they are loaded with nutrients and fiber. They are chewy and have a subtle, nutty flavor.

Wheat Berry Rice

2C	Long grain brown rice
4C	Water (or 3-1/3 if using pressure cooker)
¼C	Wheat berries
2 pinches	Sea salt

Rinse rice in water and drain. Place in a pot. Add water, sea salt, and wheat berries. Bring to a boil on high heat and then simmer on low heat for 45 minutes (or 35 minutes in a pressure cooker).

Makes 6 portions. (1 portion = 225.5 calories, 1.8 grams fat, 10% protein, 83% carbohydrates, 7% fat)

Variation: Try wild rice or quinoa instead of wheat berries.

Stovetop Rice Pilaf

1/8 C	Mild yellow onion, finely chopped
1/8 C	Green onion or shallot, finely chopped
1/8 C	Celery, chopped (about ¼" pieces)
½C	Carrots, julienned
½C	Vegetable broth
1C	Brown rice, presteamed till fluffy
½C	Wheat berries, presteamed with rice
1/8 tsp	Black ground pepper

In a large, non-stick skillet, sauté onion in 2 tablespoons of vegetable broth until tender.

Add remaining vegetable broth, heat, then add other ingredients (except celery) and sauté, stirring constantly, until carrots are hot through and slightly tender (about 5 minutes). Add celery to skillet at the very end, leaving a lot of crunch to the celery.

Add precooked rice and wheat berries to the skillet mixture, mix well while cooking a few more minutes, to blend the flavors. Fluff and serve. Makes 5 portions. (1 portion = 76.3 calories, 0.5 grams fat, 12% protein, 83% carbohydrates, 5% fat)

Wheat berries take longer to cook than does the rice, so should come out softened but still crunchy. Pilafs and stir-fries are best when they offer a variety of textures.

Baked Wild Rice Pilaf

3C	Vegetable broth or konbu broth
1 med.	Mild yellow onion, diced (about ¼ to 1/3 cup)
3 cloves	Garlic, minced
1 stalk	Celery, diced (about ½ cup)
1½ C	Fresh mushrooms, thinly sliced
1C	Wild rice
1½ tsp.	Tamari
½ tsp.	Sesame seeds, Toasted
pinch	Sea salt

To make konbu broth, soak one 3" x 3" piece of konbu in mineral water for 1 hour.

In a nonstick skillet, sauté onions, garlic, celery, and mushrooms in a little vegetable broth until onions are translucent.

Add water only if this mixture begins to stick to pan, though it shouldn't if you stir constantly and turn to medium heat.

In a saucepan, bring konbu stock to a boil. Pour into skillet with other ingredients, mix well, then place all in a casserole or baking dish.

Cover and bake at 350º F. for 1½ hours.

Remove cover and bake another 15 to 20 minutes to remove any excess liquid. Makes 3 portions. (1 portion = 264.9 calories, 1.3 grams fat, 20% protein, 76% carbohydrates, 4% fat)

Serve with a leafy green salad, for a well-rounded meal.

Stovetop Spanish Rice

1 can	Whole tomatoes, stewed (15 oz.)
½C	Green pepper, diced
1C	Water
¾C	Vegetable broth
¾C	Brown rice, Uncooked
½ tsp.	Sea salt
2 tsp.	Chili powder (or to taste)

Combine tomatoes, pepper, water, salt, and chili powder in medium saucepan. Boil over medium heat. Add rice.

Reduce heat to low, cover, and simmer until most of the liquid has been absorbed, about 45 minutes

Fluff rice, replace cover, and let stand 5 minutes before serving. Makes 4 portions. (1 portion = 174.1 calories, 1.5 grams fat, 11% protein, 82% carbohydrates, 7% fat)

You may also garnish this dish with finely diced uncooked tomatoes and green pepper, for extra texture and fresh taste. To be really creative, add a tiny bit of chopped fresh cilantro to the top of your served mounds of rice. Ole!

American Lentil Rice Pilaf

2C	Brown rice, cooked
1C	Lentils, cooked
2½ C	Water
1C	Tomatoes, ripe, chopped into small cubes
1 Medium	Onion, sliced
1 large	Celery, diced
2 stalk	Carrots, julienned
2C	Parsley, chopped
½C- ¼C	Onion, chopped
¼ tsp.	Sea salt

Sauté vegetables in tiny amount of oil for about 5 minutes.

Mix heated, cooked lentils and rice together. Stir into sautéed vegetables. Garnish with sliced tomato and parsley. Serve hot, with a wave of the flag! Makes 6 portions.

(1 portion = 166.3 calories, 1.1 grams   fat,   15% protein, 79% carbohydrates, 6% fat)

Mung Bean Surprise

1½ C	Basmati or long grain brown rice
¼C	Whole mung beans, shelled and split
1 med.	Onion, chopped
1C	Corn
1½ C	Peas and carrots, frozen
2 tsp.	Cumin
1 tsp.	Sea salt
1 tsp.	Ground cardamom
2½ C	Water
Spray	Canola oil cooking

You'll be surprised by how well all the flavors blend together in this special dish. Wash basmati rice and soak in cold water for 20 minutes. (Enriched long grain rice should not be washed.) Drain rice.

Wash split mung beans, dry, and roast in a skillet until crisp. Spray nonstick skillet with cooking spray, add onions, cumin, and sauté on moderate heat for a few seconds.

Add spices, vegetables, and salt. Stir in rice and mung beans. Add water, bring to a boil, reduce to low heat and cook about 45 minutes. For crisper vegetables, drop them into the pan after the rest has cooked for about 30 minutes, cook the dish for 15 minutes more. Let entire dish steam for 10 minutes before serving. Makes 5 portions. (1 portion = 270.4 calories, 3.790 grams fat, 10% protein, 81% carbohydrates, 9% fat)

Azuki Rice (Sekihan)

½C	Azuki beans
1¾ C	Liquid (azuki stock plus water)
1½ C	Brown or whole grain mochi (sticky) rice
½C	Brown rice

Soak all rice in cold water for 15 minutes, to soften. Rinse beans, cover with water, place in saucepan over high heat. Let beans come to a rapid boil, lower heat, and cook for 45 minutes. The cooked beans should be whole. Drain and save liquid. Put beans in a bowl to cool.

Wash rice and drain well. Measure liquid from cooked beans, add water to equal 1¾ cups of liquid. Mix rice and azuki with liquid and cook in rice cooker or in a pot. When done, turn off and let stand for 10 minutes.

Serve rice plain or garnish to taste.

Makes 6 portions. (1 portion = 277.3 calories, 0.7 grams fat, 11% protein, 8% carbohydrates, 2% fat)

*For an excellent garnish, try a mixture of salt and toasted black and white sesame seeds. To make this, mix 2 teaspoons salt with 1 tablespoon of black and white toasted sesame seeds. Serve in a small dish. A tiny spoon should be used to ladle out the salt.

Popular, Versatile Pilafs

You're probably familiar with some type of rice pilaf dish, but did you know that rice pilaf was originally a Persian dish containing rice, raisins, meats or fowl, and a sauce? These days, pilafs are a part of the cuisine all over the world. There's Spanish Rice Pilaf, Indian Saffron Rice Pilaf, and American Lentil Rice, to name only a few. Making rice pilaf is another way to easily please by presenting "gourmet" meals with little effort on your part. The trick once again is to add some chopped vegetables and spices and condiments to the rice. It's a small effort that obtains a great result.

These delicious pilaf recipes will give you some ideas, but do join in the fun and create your own. Lack of time does not need to be a problem. You can even try prepackaged pilaf mixes minus the oil and butter…very convenient.

Healthy Breakfast Alternative

We love breakfast cereals, and oatmeal or whole grain cereals are a good way to start the day. It's the milk and/or sugar we add that make breakfast less healthy for reasons we've discussed. But there's a way to enjoy whole grain cereal without sugar and dairy…and it can still be enjoyable. Simply dry-roast the grains in a hot skillet before you cook them in water. This process ("dextrinizing") will make your meal delicious. Often, simple tips like this one lead to delicious breakfasts.

Dry-roasting your grain before you cook it will give it a rich, nutty flavor.

Toasty Cooked Breakfast Cereal

1C Dry oatmeal, bulgur wheat or other breakfast whole grain.

Dry-roast grains by putting them in a nonstick skillet. Roast over a low flame or heat, shaking and tossing a little until it browns and a nice toasty aroma rises out of the pan. Then prepare as you would ordinarily.

Quinoa Fruit breakfast

1/4 cup uncooked pre-washed quinoa, or rinse well under water
1/2 cup unsweetened almond milk
1/2 teaspoon cinnamon
1/2 teaspoon vanilla extract
1 medium banana, sliced
6 strawberries, sliced
1/2 cup blueberries

Directions:
Fill a small pot of almond milk, cinnamon and vanilla, bring to a boil, reduce heat to a simmer, add quinoa, cover and cook on low until liquid evaporates, about 20 to 25 minutes. Fluff with a fork. Divide the hot quinoa in 2 bowls, top each with sliced fruit and desired toppings.

Another Versatile Crowd Pleaser

Many of us are accustomed to seeing sweet potatoes at our Thanksgiving feasts, But this family staple, steamed or mashed, because of its delicious taste and pleasing, comfort-food texture can be welcome at any meal. The sweet potato happens to be a nutrition giant as well as a crowd pleaser. It's an excellent source of vitamins C, E, the B vitamins, and high in fiber while extremely low in fat.

Sweet potatoes work well as side dishes or snacks. Try substituting three sweet potato slices for three cookies and save seven grams of fat! If you have a sweet tooth, sweet potatoes are your friend. They are filling and satisfy your sweet tooth without ruining your diet.

Steamed Sweet Potatoes or Yams

6 med.   Sweet potatoes or yams
                      Water

Place whole sweet potatoes in steamer with 1" of water and steam for approximately 15 minutes or until fork tender. Slice and serve. Or create glazed sweet potatoes by covering with the following sauce and baking for 5 more minutes. Makes 6 portions. (1 sweet potato portion = 117.0 calories, 0.125 grams fat, 7% protein, 93% carbohydrates, 1% fat) (1 yam portion = 127.8 calories, 0.1 grams fat, 5% protein, 94% carbohydrates, 1% fat) Sweet potatoes and yams are simple and simply delicious by themselves. They are great at any meal or as snacks.

Orange-Date Glaze

3C   Unsweetened orange juice
1C   Dates, pitted and blended to a mush
¼ tsp.   Vanilla
½ tsp.   Salt
½ tsp.   Corn starch
¼ tsp.   Cloves (optional)

Cook over a low flame, adding ingredients in the above order. Add corn starch last, stirring constantly as it begins to thicken. You want it to be the consistency of a thick syrup. Remove from flame and spoon over steamed yams or sweet potatoes. You can either serve directly, or place in a very hot oven and bake the flavors together for 5 minutes. Makes 6 portions. *(1 portion = 138.6 calories, 0.384 grams fat, 4% protein, 94% carbohydrates, 2% fat) (1 sweet potato portion with 1 portion orange-date glaze = 256.0 calories, 0.5 grams fat, 5% protein, 93% carbohydrates, 2% fat)*

Pasta

Whole Grain Pastas

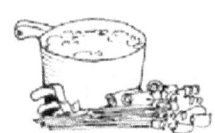

Whole grain pasta is another fast and simple way to keep your meals interesting. All you do is add some sauce, vegetables and pesto, and you have a delicious hot meal. There are so many varieties that you can experiment endlessly with the kinds of dishes you prepare. While spaghetti-type pasta is excellent, you might also try a small noodle such as vermicelli, or other common pastas such as macaroni, tortellini, corkscrew pasta - the list is endless. You can also present your dishes in colorful variety, by using green spinach pasta and orange-colored pasta, reddish pastas colored by beet juice, and so forth. Check your health food store for some possibilities.

Whole wheat pasta tastes excellent, and is also healthy. So is most Oriental pasta - for instance, buckwheat noodles. By using a variety of different pastas, you can make your dishes interesting in appearance and texture and keep your meals interesting. Another type of pasta that is gaining popularity is couscous, which is excellent as a quick hot cereal, a dressed-up entree, or in a cold salad. Try some of the recipes you'll find on the side of the box, but remember to cut out at least most of the fat if it calls even for olive oil.

Most dishes adapt well to a no-oil variation.

Couscous is a Mediterranean grain dish that most people think is a whole grain. Actually, it is a processed grain, as is pasta. Both are moderate on the EMI. But they're acceptable as entrees, and will enhance your Peace Diet so long as you remember to balance your diet with foods that are high on the EMI.

A word of caution. Most pastas are made from refined white flours, so I recommend that you use them moderately, depending on your health, because, ideally, the best grain to use is one that is not ground into flour in the first place.

Most whole grain pastas have their own instructions for preparation on the package. One simple technique is to boil the water in a pot, place the pasta in the boiling water, turn off the heat and cover pot. About 10 to 15 minutes later, depending on the thickness of the pasta, it's ready.

Tomato Vermicelli

1 tsp.	Olive oil
3 cloves	Garlic, medium-size, peeled, and minced
1 med.	Onion, chopped
1 can	Tomatoes (28 oz.), peeled, diced, undrained
1 can	Mushroom and pieces (4 oz.)
1-1/3 C	Vegetable broth, or water
1/3	Dry red wine
1 tsp.	Maple syrup or honey
¼	Cayenne pepper
½	Fresh basil (1 tsp. dried)
½ C	Fresh oregano (½ tsp. dried)
6 oz.	Vermicelli pasta, broken in halves
	Black pepper, freshly ground, to taste
dash	Sea salt

Sauté garlic and onion in olive oil, in large skillet. Add tomatoes, mushrooms, broth, wine, honey, cayenne, basil, and oregano. Bring to a boil and add the pasta. Cover and cook about 8 to 10 minutes, stirring often, until the pasta has softened. Add salt and black pepper to taste. Makes 3 portions. (3 portions = 294.8 calories, 3.5 grams fat, 17% protein, 73% carbohydrates, 10% fat)

Vegetarian Ravioli

1 bunch	Fresh spinach, chopped
1 box	Fresh mushrooms, diced ¼"
1 med.	Onion, chopped
3 cloves	Garlic, minced
1 block	Firm tofu, diced into¼" cubes
2 pkg.	Mun doo wrappers (20+)

Sauté garlic and onions in ¼ cup water
until transparent. Add mushrooms, cook approximately 3
minutes, then add spinach and continue cooking on high for 5
minutes. Add tofu and cook 3 minutes on low. Set aside and
cool.

To make raviolis, spoon tablespoonful of filling into mon
doo wrapper. Moisten edge with
water or liquid from filling and
cover with another wrapper and
press hard on edges to seal. Cook
raviolis in large pot of boiling water
for 3 minutes. Drain and serve with
marinara sauce. Makes 8 portions.
(4 portions = 135.0 calories, 1.4
grams fat, 22% protein, 68%
carbohydrates, 9% fat)

Marinara Sauce

1 round	Onion, chopped
5 cloves	Garlic, crushed
2 cans	Tomatoes (24 oz.), chopped
½C	Water
pinch	Salt or to taste
dash	White pepper
3	Fresh basil leaves or 1 tsp. dried
½ C	Cilantro, chopped

Water-sauté garlic. Add ½ can water and simmer 30 to 60 minutes. Makes 12 portions. (1 portion = 19.2 calories, 0.2 grams fat, 16% protein, 76% carbohydrates, 8% fat)

Pasta With Eggplant Sauce

This is a great main dish for any gathering. Leftover sauce can be used over brown rice for lunch the next day.

½ tsp.	Olive oil
1½ lb.	Eggplant, unpeeled and in ½" chunks
1 large	Red onion, chopped
3 large	Garlic cloves, minced
1C	Mushrooms, coarsely chopped
1C	Green peppers, coarsely chopped
2-3 cans	Plum tomatoes (1 lb.)
2 tsp.	Dry basil
1 tsp.	Dry oregano
1 tsp.	Sugar
2/3 C	Cilantro
	Salt, to taste
	Pepper, to taste
1 lb.	Pasta

Heat oil, add eggplant, onions, and sauté over medium heat until soft and lightly browned, stirring frequently. Add garlic, mushrooms, and bell pepper, and continue to sauté. Add tomatoes, basil, oregano, and sugar. Cook covered for 10 minutes. Add cilantro. Season with salt and pepper. Cover and simmer 15 to 20 minutes.

Cook pasta. Pour hot pasta sauce over pasta and serve. Makes 6 to 8 portions. (1 portion = 265.5 calories, 2.0 grams fat, 19% protein, 75% carbohydrates, 7% fat)

Pasta with Roasted Vegetables

12	Plum tomatoes, quartered lengthwise
1 lb.	Asparagus, trimmed 1 Zucchini, quartered
2	Yellow crooked- neck squash, quartered
1 head	Broccoli, cut in bite-size pieces
2	Long eggplant or 1 round eggplant, peeled
1 basket	Mushrooms, cut in halves
1 small	Garlic head
2 tsp.	Fresh lemon juice
1 Tbsp.	Fresh basil
1 Tbsp.	Fresh cilantro
	Salt to taste
1 lb.	Pepper to taste Pasta of choice

Seat oven rack in lower third of oven. Preheat oven to 450° F. Cut asparagus, zucchini, yellow crooked-neck squash and eggplant in 2" lengths.

In large roasting pan, toss vegetables with olive oil and garlic. Roast 20 minutes until vegetables are tender.

In large pot of boiling water, cook pasta until tender but firm, about 8 minutes. Drain and transfer to roasting pan and toss gently to combine with vegetables. Serve immediately. Makes 8 to 10 portions. (1 portion = 233.7 calories, 2.1 grams fat, 18% protein, 74% carbohydrates, 8% fat)

Bow Tie Pasta With Miso Sauce

1 lb.	Bow tie (Farfalle) pasta, cooked and drained
1	Red bell pepper, julienned
1	Green bell pepper, julienned
1 small	Red onion, diced
1 sm. Head	Broccoli, cut in florets and blanched
1 small	Zucchini, diced and blanched
2 Tbsp.	Olive oil
4	Green onions, sliced
2 cloves	Garlic, minced
¼C	Light miso
1-1½ C	Veggie broth, warm
¼C	Parsley, chopped
¼ tsp.	Pepper flakes (or more to taste)

Put cooked pasta in a large mixing bowl.

Add bell peppers, onion, broccoli, and zucchini.

In a medium skillet over medium heat, sauté green onions and garlic in oil for 1 to 2 minutes. Add miso, stir. Stir in veggie broth. Add parsley and pepper flakes. Pour over pasta and toss. Makes 12 to 14 portions. (1 portion = 93.2 calories, 2.9 grams fat, 15% protein, 58% carbohydrates, 27% fat)

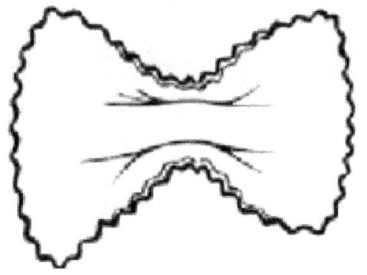

Asian Cold Pasta

Cold pasta dishes can be healthy, but be careful. A 1-cup serving of cold pasta salad can be as high as 24 grams fat and 51% of 420 calories? (Kraft® Herb and Garlic Pasta Salad).

The reason cold pasta dishes, such as pasta salads, can be high in fat is the oil used in the dressing. Oil of all kinds is the most concentrated source of calories at 9 calories per gram. One solution is to use nonfat dressings or an Asian dipping sauce. They can be delicious this way and can be used as an entrée, a side dish, or they may form the base of a salad. The cooking process may be a bit different from the pastas you're used to cooking, so read the instructions carefully.

To make cold noodle dishes, drain the noodles when they're cooked. Immerse them in ice cold water quickly (don't soak), drain, then prepare the rest of your dish.

Asian cold noodles are often eaten by dipping them into a delicious sauce. Seasoned rice vinegar, soy sauces, and other novel taste treats can be used. Prepared dipping sauces can also be found wherever Asian foods are sold.

To further enhance these dishes, you can also add cold vegetables of your own choosing. Asian vegetables will give you a nice break from routine. Sliced vegetables are especially good with cold noodle dishes. Choose your own combinations, and you'll soon be learning the secrets that it took Asian chefs centuries to perfect.

Two excellent suggestions are cold soba (cooked according to directions on package, then cooled in refrigerator) with soy sauce; and cold somen, also cooked according to package, dressed up with shredded cabbage, cold azuki beans, and thinly sliced cucumber, with a tablespoon of rice wine vinegar drizzled over the combination. Delicious.

Try cold soba or cold somen noodles with a dip sauce as a side dish.

Basic Buckwheat Noodles

Buckwheat noodles are one of my favorite pasta dishes. This is one whole grain pasta that is commonly served even in restaurants. At Japanese restaurants, it is served hot or cold. It's also an excellent basic cereal grain product around which to plan a meal.

1 pkg.	Buckwheat (soba) noodle
1 Tbsp.	Green onion, chopped
1	Japanese soba sauce
	(can or bottle) or prepare dip sauce
	below Nori flakes (optional)

Boil enough water to immerse the noodles in a pot, and place the noodles in the boiling water. As it boils, it will foam so before it overflows, pour a small amount of cool water into the saucepan and the foaming will stop for a short while and will build up again. You'll have to do this about three times before it is cooked. If noodles already contain salt, do not salt cooking water. If they do not contain salt, a pinch of sea salt can be added to the cooking water.

After the noodles are cooked, drain and rinse in cool water and drain again.

Garnish with green onion and nori flakes. Serve cold. Use the following sauce for flavor as a dipping sauce. Makes 3 portions. (1 portion = 281.3 calories, 1.0 grams fat, 19% protein, 78% carbohydrates, 3% fat)

Asian Dipping Sauce

¼C	Low-sodium soy sauce (for the simplest sauce you can just use soy sauce)
2C	Water
1 piece	Konbu (about 3" x 2")
1 tsp.	Ginger, grated

Boil the konbu in water for 5 minutes; remove the konbu (it can be sliced and eaten with other vegetables) and add the other ingredients. You can vary the taste of the sauce by adding the ingredients below.

1 tsp.	Wasabi (Japanese horseradish, the kind used on sushi)
1-2 tsp.	Lemon juice for a tangy taste
1 clove	Garlic, crushed

Serve in separate bowls for each person to dip their noodles. You can make several servings of this recipe, and keep some on hand in the refrigerator to use on quick-cooked Asian noodles when you're in the mood. Makes 8 portions (2 cups). (1 portion = 5.0 calories, 0.0 grams fat, 35% protein, 64% carbohydrates, 2% fat)

Buckwheat Noodle Medley

1 pkg.	Buckwheat (8-10 oz. soba) noodles
1 Tbsp.	Fresh ginger, grated
	Water to cool noodles while cooking
	Low-sodium soy sauce, to taste
	Any leftover vegetables or beans, especially broccoli, peas, beans, cabbage, collards, kale, mustard greens, spinach, turnip greens

Prepare noodles as above, then cool.

In large bowl or pan, combine noodles, grated fresh ginger, and small amount of low-sodium soy sauce or tamari. Then cut lightly-cooked vegetables (anything you choose to use) into bite-size pieces.

Toss together with cold soba, and serve.

Makes 3 portions. (1 portion = 279.6 calories, 1.0 grams fat, 17% protein, 80% carbohydrates, 3% fat)

Asian Pasta Salad

½ lb.	Buckwheat noodles
1C	Yellow zucchini, julienne
1	Carrot, shredded
1C	Celery, diced
1C	Daikon (Japanese turnip), diced
2 Tbsp.	Lemon juice
1 Tbsp.	Umeboshi plum paste
3	Scallions, minced(green part only)
½ can	Olives, sliced

Cook buckwheat noodles according to directions. Cool. Cook, cool, and julienne zucchini and set aside. Shred carrot, set aside. Blend lemon juice, umeboshi, and scallions into a dressing. Toss pasta with the vegetables and dressing. Garnish with parsley. Makes 5 portions. (1 portion = 196.9 calories, 2.5 grams fat, 14% protein, 75% carbohydrates, 10% fat)

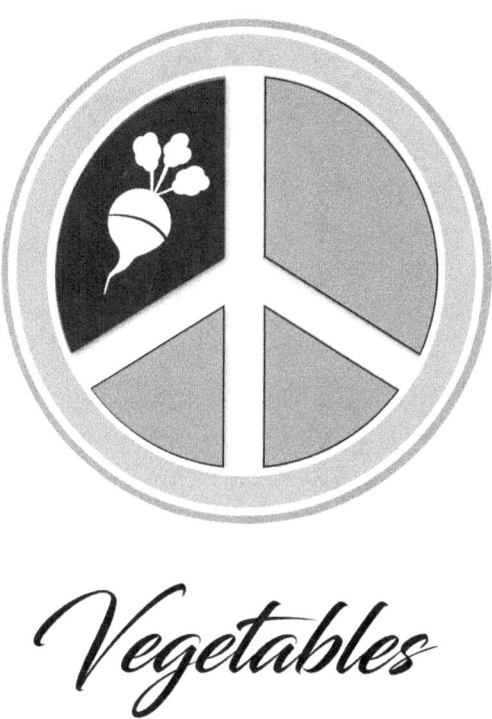

Vegetables

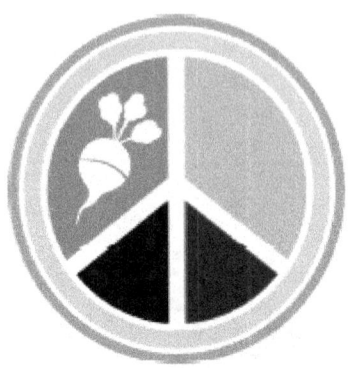

VEGETABLES

Vegetables are nutrition powerhouses; thus, they are essential to the Peace Diet. It's no accident that there's an abundance of wonderful vegetable recipes in this book. Vegetables have the highest rating on the SMI scale, and you should try to eat at least seven to eleven servings per day. Fresh vegetables have the highest nutritive value, followed by frozen and finally by canned.

Both raw and cooked vegetables have nutritional strong points, so it's to your benefit to use both. Using both raw and cooked vegetables gives you not only better protection but also variety. Raw vegetables and juices are recognized around the world not just for their nutritional value but also for their curative value. It is widely believed that five servings of fruits and vegetables per day are associated with lower risk of stroke, obesity and obesity-related diseases, and even aging and degenerative diseases.

Our recipes will cover cooked, raw, and soup vegetables. First, let's take a look at cooked vegetables.

Less Oil, Better Nutrition

A valuable tip is to avoid cooking with oil to whatever extent possible, which is most of the time. For instance, a one-cup serving of vegetables sautéed in oil can have as much as 42% of the calories from fat – which greatly diminishes the overall nutritional value of the dish. This isn't necessary since other ways of cooking work as well and can offer just as much flavor. One way is to use a nonstick ceramic skillet and sauté with water. For more flavor, sauté with canned vegetable broth or a vegetarian powder and water mix.

For more flavor, you can sauté with a little wine or try sautéing a small amount of onion and garlic in the vegetable broth before you add the other ingredients. You will never miss the oil, but you will reap the benefits.

Salads and Dressings

Salads are super high on the SMI scale. They're one of the easiest and tastiest ways to eat your high-SMI foods. If you enjoy a salad as a main course for lunch or dinner, you can get your daily requirement of vegetables all at once. Since salads often consist of all raw foods, they have a natural balance of fiber, nutrients, and water that your body needs. While cooking food can deplete vitamins, destroy enzymes that help digestion, and even damage fats and proteins, this does not happen to salads, which are raw food in its natural state. They have no processed foods or additives to worry about.

However, there is one key problem. Most people ruin their salads before they take their first bite by dousing them with oily, high-fat salad dressings. Oily salad dressings are the lowest in SMI of all foods. They'll instantly ruin the weight-loss value of a salad. The trick is to use salad dressings that are medium to high in SMI and contain little or no oil. This is not hard to do with a little work, as you will see in the section below on salad dressings.

Besides using medium to high SMI dressings, you can choose to try different types of salads that don't rely quite so heavily on the dressing. There are many of varieties: corn salads, beet salads, three-bean salads and others that will delight your taste buds without tempting you to resort to high-fat dressings. Some cold noodle dishes also adapt well to salad recipes. Or you can modify the following to create your own.

Mark Ellman's Tomato Miso Vinaigrette

Tomato miso vinaigrette was probably the favorite dressing on the Hawaii Health Program. You will enjoy the Pacific Rim tastes of this dressing, too.

2 Tbsp.	Onion, chopped
1C	White wine
1/2 tsp.	Garlic, chopped
2	sprigs Tarragon (fresh)
1C	Rice vinegar
1C	Tomato purée
8 Tbsp.	Red miso
1 tsp.	Sesame seed oil
3 tsp.	Extra virgin olive oil

Sauté onion and garlic in wine. Reduce to a glacé.

Add vinegar and reduce by one-half. Add tomato and tarragon. Reduce by one-half and add red miso. Boil once. Emulsify in blender with olive oil and fresh tarra- gon, with a touch of sesame seed oil. Add water if too thick.

Makes 24 portions.   (1 portion = 31 calories, 1.1 grams fat, 14% protein, 49% carbohydrates, 37% fat)

Chinese Lettuce Wraps

Any type of green lettuce leaves---cut/break into nice shapes for wrapping (green, red, butter, small romaine leaves, or manoa lettuce are the best to use).

Filling

1 cup	round onions chopped small but not minced
2 cloves	minced or pressed garlic
2 tspn	grated ginger
2 Tbsp	soy sauce

(For more flavor, season with mushroom powder as desired if adding more ingredients.)

2 Tblspn	pure maple syrup
I Tbsp	mirin (sweet japanese rice wine vinegar)
1 small can	water chestnuts, drained and finely chopped
1 large can	bamboo strips, drained, rinsed, and chopped
1 cup	chopped mushrooms
1 Tblspn	ground sesame seeds (optional)
	Chopped cilantro (optional)

Thinly sliced green onions (optional)
Minced celery (optional)
(Don't make mixture too salty since you will be adding soy dressing w/wrap.)
1 cup "ground round" style seitan (wheat gluten)
(more seitan can be added for larger serving)
Note: If seitan is not available, use Mrs. Chen's baked tofu or any other brand of baked tofu (chop/add quantity desired). Meatless Ground (NonGMO Soy from COSTCO) can also be used (comes in green box).

Start off by sauteing onions, ginger, and garlic in a few teaspoons of sesame oil. If too dry, add a few teaspoons of water (a little at a time instead of using too much oil). Add chopped mushrooms and keep stirring to cook. Then add chestnuts and bamboo shoots. Keep sautéing and then add soy sauce, maple syrup, and mirin, stirring completely (adjust your heat). When everything looks cooked, add the seitan or baked tofu last. Sprinkle sesame seeds---keep stirring until done. Place in large serving bowl. Sprinkle thinly sliced green onions and then more sesame seeds on top before serving with lettuce.

Soy dressing (to drizzle on to filling to be wrapped in lettuce):

Mix together 2 Tblspn brown rice vinegar, 3 Tblspn maple syrup, 1 Tblspn mirin,3/4 Cup soy sauce, 2 tspn minced/or pressed garlic.
Add to taste, minced/mashed green chili peppers (about a teaspoon).

Note: Hawaiian green chili peppers seem to have the best flavor when adding to soy sauce dressings. Buy a small handful (from Chinatown okay) and freeze it for future use (since you probably will use only one chili pepper at a time).

Thousand Island Dressing

No, this is not the usual high fat version! This one is so good that many people believe that it is "illegal," but when you see that the fat content is less than one gram per serving you'll want to use it more often.

1/4 C	Water
1/8 tsp.	Salt
1/8 tsp.	Pepper
1 tsp.	Seasoned salt
2 Tbsp.	Tomato ketchup
1C	Tofu (soft), crumbled
4 sprigs	Parsley (fresh) (optional)
1 Tbsp.	Cucumber, chopped fine
1 Tbsp.	Celery chopped fine or pickle relish

Whiz all ingredients, except cucumber, celery, or pickle relish, in blender. Add cucumber, celery, or pickle relish. Chill and serve.

Makes 12 portions (about 1-1/2 cups). (1 portion = 18 calories, 0.8 gram fat, 34% protein, 26% carbohydrates, 40% fat)

Great Caesar Salad

The traditional Caesar Salad can be a fine meal in itself, and is often mixed and tossed at tableside in American, French, and Italian restaurants with great panache. You can serve this to guests, with a flourish, or keep the secret to yourself. But whatever you do, rest assured that this version eliminates the anchovies and raw egg — two possibly problematic ingredients in the traditional version of this dish. Most of the fatty olive oil is also eliminated from the dressing. In the process, the taste is actually improved! So enjoy this traditional treat, especially on those evenings when you're too tired to cook but know you deserve something special.

SALAD INGREDIENTS:

1 head	Endive, trimmed
1 head	Red leaf lettuce, torn into pieces
1/4 C	Arugula (also called Rocket), torn to pieces
	Radicchio (a small-leaf Mediterranean lettuce)
1/4 C	Oil-free croutons (low-fat, store-bought)
1/2 C	Black pepper, ground, to taste

There are many excellent low-fat Caesar Salad dressings on the shelves of your health food store. Or, if you have time and want something special, make your own, as follows. If you like the addition of a splash of sherry but don't have time to make your own dressing, just add a tablespoonful to your bottled salad dressing and mix well before using. A very nice touch!

Great Caesar Salad Dressing

2 Tbsp.	Roasted garlic
1/4 C	Sherry cooking wine
1 tsp.	Lemon juice (fresh)
1 tsp.	Salt, to taste
1 tsp.	Extra virgin olive oil
1/4 tsp.	Rosemary (fresh), minced
1 Tbsp.	Dijon mustard
1 tsp.	A.1.® Steak Sauce
Dash	Tabasco®, to taste

Toss greens, then dress with store-bought dressing.
Or, if making your own dressing (above), pre-mix salad dressing by whisking ingredients together in a bowl. Set aside. Mix and toss salad, chill, add dressing and dust with pepper just before serving. Excellent with a side of garlic bread. Makes 2 portions as an entrée and 4 portions as side dish. (1 entrée portion = 154 calories, 3.2 grams fat, 16% protein, 61% carbohydrates, 23% fat) (1 side dish portion = 77 calories, 1.6 grams fat, 16% protein, 61% carbohydrates, 23% fat)

Miso Potato Salad

This dish combines Japanese and American cuisine into a blend that perfectly illustrates what is unique and delicious about Island food. This dish saves well when refrigerated. You can make it at home and take to the office to really dress up your lunch. This potato salad is full of flavor but without the high-fat content of mayonnaise. A tablespoon of mayonnaise contains 99 calories and 11 grams of fat while a tablespoon of miso is 35 calories and only 1 gram of fat. This is a fast and healthy alternative to other potato salads.

1 large	Russet potato
2 Tbsp.	Red miso paste
1 Tbsp.	Sweet pickle juice
2 Tbsp.	Sweet pickles, minced fine
1/4 tsp.	Mustard (prepared, not dry)

Microwave whole, scrubbed potato on high, for about 4 minutes, or until easy to pierce with a fork. Remove, cool in freezer for 1 minute. In the meantime mix all other ingredients in a bowl.
Remove potato from freezer and chop into 1/2" cubes. Mix with other ingredients, mashing slightly if you wish to provide variety in texture.

Makes 1 portion. (1 portion = 257 calories, 2.3 grams fat, 11% protein, 81% carbohydrates, 8% fat)

Peter Merriman's Mixed Green Vegetable Salad with Ka'u Gold® Potatoes

3-4 oz.	Summer greens
1 lb.	Ka'u Gold®or Yukon Gold® potatoes or other white potatoes
1	Maui onion, sliced
21/2 lb.	Broccoli, minced fine
1	Pineapple (fresh), cut into chunks

Dijon Vinaigrette (use as much as you need) Wash and boil potatoes until tender. Soak in cold water. Peel and cut into cubes.

Wash summer greens and drain thoroughly. Lay in a salad bowl.

Mix cubed potatoes, onion, broccoli, pineapple and Dijon Vinaigrette. Place on summer greens and serve immediately.

DIJON VINAIGRETTE DRESSING:

1 box	Mori Nu Tofu®
1/3 C	Grey Poupon® Dijon mustard
1/3 C	Red wine vinegar
1/4 tsp.	Black pepper, ground

Place all ingredients in a food processor and blend until smooth. Place in a covered container and store in refrigerator for up to 1 week.

Makes 8 portions. (1 portion = 130 calories, 1.6 grams fat, 13% protein, 76% carbohydrates, 11% fat)

Carrot-Celery-Pepper Sticks & Garden Dip

Using dips with vegetables makes eating raw or cooked vegetables more fun. This dip is a good example. Another great dip is the hummus found in my original Dr. Shintani's Eat More, Weigh Less Diet book on page 235.

VEGETABLES:

4 Large	Carrots
1	Green bell pepper
4 sticks	Celery

Other vegetables of choice. Peel carrots, cut into more or less uniform strips. Cut celery similarly. Core pepper, cut into similar-sized strips. Plate on crudité tray, or plate. In the center, put a bowl of Garden Dip. You may also serve flowerettes of broccoli and cauliflower.

GARDEN DIP:

1C	Green peas (frozen and thawed, or canned), drained
1/4 C	Avocado
1/4 C	Green onion, chopped fine
	Salt and pepper, to taste
1/8 C	Water
1 clove	Garlic, minced

Blend all ingredients until creamy. Garnish with pimientos, for color.
Makes 8 portions. (1 portion = 49 calories, 1.1 grams fat, 14% protein, 66% carbohydrates, 19% fat)

Lomi Tomato

This is a vegetarian version of "Lomi Salmon" which is a standard modern Hawaiian lu'au food. People are surprised how good this is, but they shouldn't be. Why? Because these days there is often not much salmon in the Lomi Salmon anyway and people still like it. So, why not try it without the salmon and thus eliminate the cholesterol.

5	Tomatoes, diced
8	Green onions, thinly sliced
1 medium	Onion, finely chopped
1-2 Tbsp.	Cider vinegar
1 tsp.	Hawaiian salt
3-5 drops	Tabasco® sauce

Combine all ingredients and chill thoroughly.

Makes 8 portions. (1 portion = 23 calories, 0.2 gram fat, 15% protein, 78% carbohydrates, 7% fat)

Fragrant Salad

This is a variation on a Japanese favorite - vinegared vegetables ("namasu"). Just mix together, then dress to taste with salt and mirin, a widely available form of alcohol-free, thick sake. 5 medium Radishes, scrubbed and grated fine

1 large	Cucumber, scrubbed and sliced to 1" coins
1/4 C	Cabbage, grated
2 Tbsp.	Lemon peel, grated
3 Tbsp.	Lemon juice
1/2 tsp.	Salt, or to taste
1/2 Tbsp.	Maple syrup

Mirin, to taste. Mix lemon juice and maple syrup in a small bowl.

Set aside. In a serving bowl, toss together vegetables and lemon peel. Dress with lemon juice and maple syrup mixture, add salt and mirin.

Makes 4 portions. (1 portion = 24 calories, 0.2 gram fat, 9% protein, 87% carbohydrates, 5% fat)

Summer Relish Salad

1	Red bell pepper, diced coarsely
1 small	Zucchini squash, chopped
1C	Corn (fresh), steamed lightly then scraped from cob
1C	Red onion, chopped
2 Tbsp.	Mint (fresh), chopped
1/8 tsp.	Salt
2 Tbsp.	Balsamic vinegar

Combine all ingredients in a small bowl, then serve.

Makes 2 generous portions. (1 portion = 116 calories, 0.5 gram fat, 14% protein, 83% carbohydrates, 4% fat)

Green Bean Salad

1C	Green beans (canned or cooked), drained
1/2 head	Lettuce, broken into bite-sized pieces
1C	Tomatoes, chopped
1C	Onions, diced

Salad dressing of choice (low fat) Toss all ingredients together, then dress and serve.

Makes 4 portions. (1 portion = 49 calories, 1.1 grams fat, 15% protein, 66% carbohydrates, 19% fat)

Asparagus Artichoke Salad

1/2 C	Marinated artichoke hearts (bottled), rinse off oil
1 pkg.	Asparagus, 8-oz. frozen and thawed, drained well
1/2 C	Red onion, chopped
1C	Red bib lettuce, torn into bite-sized shreds
1 sm. can	Pickled beet slices, drained, juice reserved
1/2 C	Beet juice from pickled beets
2 Tbsp.	Balsamic vinegar
1 tsp.	A.1.® Steak Sauce
	Salt, to taste
	Black pepper, freshly ground, to taste

Mix last three ingredients into a dressing, toss all other ingredients together, then dress and serve.

Makes 4 portions.

Green Papaya Salad

1 clove	Garlic
2	Hawaiian chili peppers
1/2 lb.	Green papaya, peeled, seeded, and shredded
1	Tomato, sliced
2 Tbsp.	Thai fish sauce (optional)
3 Tbsp.	Lime juice
	Sugar, to taste
1 head	Lettuce or cabbage, shredded

Grind garlic and chili peppers.

Combine shredded papaya, sliced tomato, fish sauce, lime juice and pepper-garlic mixture and mix well.

Serve on a bed of lettuce or cabbage.

A little sugar will sweeten the tartness of this popular Thai salad.

Makes 4-6 portions (5 cups). (1 portion = 48 calories, 0.3 grams fat, 16% protein, 78% carbohydrates, 5% fat)

Fresh Citrus Salad

This is an excellent breakfast or quick-lunch dish, especially when served with a side of cinnamon toast.

2	Kiwi fruit, peeled and sliced
2	Bananas, cut into 1" coins
1/2	Papaya, halved, seeded, peeled, and cubed
2 tsp.	Lime zest
1 Tbsp.	Green onion with stems, finely chopped
1 tsp.	Lime juice (fresh)

Mix all fruits together, then mix all other ingredients and whisk, to use for dressing. Add dressing just before serving.

Makes 4 portions as an entrée, 6 portions as a side dish. (1 entrée portion = 99 calories, 0.5 grams fat, 5% protein, 91% carbohydrates, 4% fat) (1 side dish portion = 66 calories, 0.4 grams fat, 5% protein, 91% carbohydrates, 4% fat)

Soups

Soups have always been the way to get a lot of ingredients – and a lot of nutrition – into one pot at one time, tasty and easy to make. Plant-based soups are no exception; in fact, it's even truer for them. A bowl of soup, a slice of whole-grain bread, and a piece of fruit for dessert – Voila! A feast.

One of the best tasting soups is almost an "instant" soup. Basmati may be the King of Rice, but miso is the Queen of Soups. In fact, the two can make a perfect match in a variety of menus.

Miso is made from fermented soybean paste. It is a traditional Japanese soup base that has served Asian chefs well for centuries. Deliciously robust, highly nutritious, this soup stock is simple and easy to prepare. Today, miso can be found in supermarkets and in health food stores. You can also find various types of miso in Oriental food stores. More and more people are appreciating and seeking out Asian foods.

ALMOST INSTANT: To make basic miso soup (Zip Miso Soup), boil water and just before serving dissolve some miso in it, as described below. Make sure it is blended smoothly to get the lumps out. Garnish it with some chopped green onions or seaweed, and it's ready to serve. For one variety of miso soup, simply prepare some of your favorite vegetables in water. Just before you serve them, dissolve the miso into the hot water, and you've created a delicious miso-based soup. Miso is very high in protein, so it is a great substitute for any animal product-based soup. It is also quite high in sodium. However, this can be controlled by the amount of miso you use per cup of hot water.

For Some Variety, Try...

Miso cam be used to season all types of soups, and it can flavor and add nutrition to sauces, gravies, salad dressings, dips, casseroles, and vegetables...it can even be used as a marinade.

Try miso soup for breakfast or with dinner.

Try the following miso recipes for a variation that will satisfy your appetite for something special.

Peking Hot & Sour Soup

2 tsp.	Cornstarch
2 Tbsp.	Cider vinegar
1 can	Vegetable broth with 1-1/2 cup water
1 Tbsp.	Soy sauce (low sodium)
1/2 C	Water
1/2 tsp.	Sea salt
1/4 C	Wood ears (dried black fungus)
1/4 C	Golden needles (dried lily flowers)
1/4 C	Tofu, cubed (about 1/2 small cake)
1/4 tsp.	White ground pepper
1 Tbsp.	Scallions, minced (garnish)

Boil water and soak wood ears and golden needles separately for about 15 minutes. Break off hard pieces from wood ears and hard stems from golden needles, if any. Cut golden needles in halves and snap the large pieces of wood ears into smaller pieces. Wash and drain.

Mix the cornstarch with 1/2 cup cold water. Stir until smooth. Mix vinegar and pepper.
Mix vegetable broth and water. Add salt and soy sauce. Bring to a boil and add wood ears and golden needles. Boil 1 minute. Add tofu. As soup boils, stir in the well-stirred cornstarch mixture until it thickens. Serve in bowl with vinegar and pepper. Garnish with scallions. Serve Hot.

Makes 4 to 6 portions. (1 portion = 47 calories, 1.2 grams fat, 30% protein, 48% carbohydrates, 21% fat)

Potato and Corn Chowder

Probably the best liked soup on the Hawaii Health Program.

2 tsp.	Dry cooking sherry
1-1/4 C	Sweet yellow onion, finely chopped
2 cloves	Garlic, crushed
2C	Red potatoes, cubed
1 can	Vegetable stock (14-1/4 oz.)
1C	Soy milk
1C	Corn kernels (fresh or frozen)
1	Bay leaf
1/4 tsp.	Paprika
1/4 tsp.	Thyme
1 tsp.	Basil
	Salt, to taste
	Pepper, to taste
	Olive oil cooking spray

Add wine to a large oil-sprayed skillet and heat. Add onions and garlic and sauté for 5 minutes, stirring frequently to prevent browning. Add water as needed.
Add potatoes, bay leaf, herbs, and stock to sautéed onions and garlic. Cover pan, bring to a boil, and cook over medium heat for 10 to 15 minutes. When the potatoes are tender, add the corn and milk. Simmer until the corn is tender, about 3 minutes. Discard the bay leaf. Use your hand blender to partially purée the mixture, or remove a cup of soup and purée in blender or food processor, then return it to the pot. This will give your soup a creamy texture. Season with salt and/or pepper to taste.

Makes 6 to 8 portions. (1 portion = 117 calories, 1.3 grams fat, 18% protein, 70% carbohydrates, 10% fat)

This and other cream soups are a snap to make if you have a hand blender. With this, you can partially blend the soup right in the pot. Just wait until it's almost done then do your blending, leaving enough chunky ingredients to give the soup texture. Watch out for spattering though, if it's really hot.

Corn Soup

This corn soup is especially delicious and a variation of it was served at one of the follow-up sessions of the Governor's group. People liked it so much that they were getting seconds from the kitchen before it ran out.

6 ears	Corn (fresh), husked, silk removed or substitute two packages cut corn (10 oz., frozen), thawed
1 Tbsp.	Water
2 medium	Tomatoes, peeled, and coarsely chopped
1 medium	Onion, finely chopped
1 Tbsp.	Cumin, ground
3 cloves	Garlic, peeled and minced
1	Green pepper, seeds reserved, deribbed, and cubed
1	Red pepper, seeds reserved, deribbed, and cubed
1 tsp.	Lite Salt® (optional)
4 cups	Vegetable broth

GARNISH:

Jalapeño pepper, seeded and minced
Cilantro (fresh)
Strips of roasted pimento

Cut the kernels from the ears of corn over a bowl to catch any corn milk. Then scrape the ears with the back of a knife to extract the remaining milk. The milk will act as a natural thickener for the soup.

Heat the water in a heavy casserole over low heat. Add the tomato, onion, and cumin. Cook, stirring, until the onion is softened, but not brown. Add the garlic and stir for about 2 minutes. Add the peppers and optional Lite Salt®. Continue stirring until the peppers are slightly limp. Add the stock and corn milk and, stirring, bring to a simmer. Cook 5 minutes, so the corn is still crunchy. Taste for seasonings.

To finish, garnish with cilantro leaves, strips of pimento, and a sprinkle of Jalapeño pepper. For a thick- er consistency, thicken with cornstarch and water. Serve hot.

Makes 8 servings.   (1 portion = 106 calories, 1.1 grams fat, 17% protein, 74% carbohydrates, 9% fat)

Wakame Soup

3C	Water
2 cloves	Garlic, sliced
1 medium	Onion, chopped
1 medium	Carrot, chopped fine 1 medium Potato, chopped fine
1 oz.	Wakame (fresh), wash and chop into small pieces
4"x4"	Konbo (seaweed), soaked
3	Shiitake mushroom

In a saucepan, soak konbo and shiitake mushrooms in 3 cups of cold water for 1/2 hour to make broth. Add garlic, onion, carrot, potato, and wakame to the broth and boil.

Makes 6 portions. (1 portion = 39 calories, 0.2 gram fat, 11% protein, 85% carbohydrates, 4% fat)

Wakame Onion Mushroom Soup

1 handful	Wakame
1	Onion, diced
4C	Water
1-2 Tbsp.	Miso
2	Shiitake mushrooms (dried)

Soak wakame and mushrooms in 1 cup of water
until soft, cut into 1" pieces. Sauté onions in 1/4 cup of water.
Add water from soaked wakame and mushrooms and the rest of
the water. Bring to a boil, add the wakame and mushrooms, and
cook over low flame until it is tender. Add miso to taste by
diluting 1 to 2 tablespoons of miso in a ladle full of the soup
water, mashing and smoothing out the miso and adding it back to
the pot. Leftover grain or noodles may be added if desired.

Makes 6 portions.   (1 portion = 23 calories, 0.3 grams
fat, 16% protein, 73% carbohydrates, 12% fat)

Variations:
Other variations on this soup would include adding onions,
cauliflower, shiitake mushrooms, celery, tofu chunks, etc., to
wakame broth. You can also add medi- um grain brown rice, or
barley, or use miso soup as a broth to pour over your whole
grains.

Wheat Berry Vegetable Soup

1C	Kidney beans (dried), soaked overnight in water and drained
2 tsp.	Olive oil
1 large	Onion, chopped
1 large	Leek, washed well and chopped
1 stalk	Celery, chopped
1C	Wheat berries, soaked overnight in water and drained
1 medium	Potato, peeled and diced
1-1/2 C	Tomatoes (canned), chopped
3 sprigs	Rosemary (fresh), about 3" long, tied in cheesecloth

Bring beans and 3 cups water to a boil in a medium, covered saucepan. Lower heat and simmer until beans are tender, about 40 minutes to 1 hour.

Heat oil in a separate large saucepan over medium- high heat. Reduce heat to medium-low and add onion, leek, and celery.

Sauté, stirring often until soft, about 10 minutes. Stir in beans and cooking water. Add wheat berries, potato, tomato, and rosemary sprigs. Cover and simmer gently over low heat until wheat berries are swol- len and tender (about 40 minutes). Stir occasionally to keep vegetables from sticking. Remove rosemary and discard. Good hot or cold. Freezes well.

Makes 6 portions.   (1 portion = 224 calories, 2.5 grams fat, 16% protein, 75% carbohydrates, 9% fat)

Mushroom-Broccoli Noodle Soup

1 medium	Onion, cut into thin crescents
2 oz.	Mushrooms (dried), soaked and sliced
1 medium	Broccoli bunch, stem cut in quarter rounds and flowerettes cut into
2" pieces	
1 can	Water chestnuts, sliced (8 oz., 5 oz. drained)
6C	Water, boiling
2C	Vegetable broth
1/4 tsp.	Sea salt
2C	Soba noodles
2 Tbsp.	Sesame seeds, lightly toasted

2-3 Tbsp. Soy sauce or tamari (low sodium) In a skillet, water sauté onions until transparent. If they begin to stick, add more water, as necessary. Add broccoli stems, sauté briefly, then add mushrooms, water chestnuts, boiling water, vegetable broth, and sea salt. Cover and bring to a boil, then lower heat and simmer for 10 minutes. Add noodles and simmer for a few minutes, until tender. Add broccoli flowerettes, cook until bright green, about 1 minute. Sprinkle sesame seeds onto soup broth. Add soy sauce. Stir and heat, without boiling, until done to taste.

Makes 10 portions.   (1 portion = 78 calories, 1.1 grams fat, 20% protein, 68% carbohydrates, 12% fat)

Breakfast Miso Soup

2½ C	Water
1	Wakame seaweed (3" strip)
1/8 C	Firm tofu, chopped to ½" chunks
1	Green onion, with stems, chopped fine
1 Tbsp.	Barley miso

Bring water to a boil, add wakame and one-half of green onion, simmer 5 minutes.

Turn off heat, add miso to taste by diluting 1 to 2 tablespoons of miso in a ladle full of the soup water, mashing and smoothing out the miso and adding it back to the pot.

Pour into a large bowl, over small chunks of tofu. Garnish with chopped green onions, serve steaming hot.

Makes 4 to 6 portions. (1 portion = 18.1 calories, 0.8 grams fat, 30% protein, 34% carbohydrates, 35% fat)

Cream of Broccoli Soup

5C	Vegetable broth
1½ C	Broccoli, both tops and stems, but separated, chopped
1 small	Yellow onion, diced
1½ C	Brown rice, cooked or leftover oatmeal
1 Tbsp.	White or barley miso

Boil broth or water, add broccoli stems and onion. Cover and simmer for 10 minutes.

Put 2 cups of the soup liquid in the blender with rice or oatmeal, blend until smooth, then return to the pot. Add broccoli tops and simmer briefly, until they're tender. Flavor with miso to taste and serve. Makes 6 to 8 portions. (1 portion =86.9 calories, 0.8 grams fat, 21% protein, 71% carbohydrates, 7% fat)

Portuguese Bean Soup

6 cloves	Garlic, crushed
1½	Round onions, chopped
2 stalks	Celery, chopped
4	Carrots, diced
1 can	Vegetable broth (14½ oz.)
2 cans	Whole tomatoes plus juice (large), cut in chunks
3	Potatoes, cubed
3C	Beans, cooked
½ head	Cabbage, chopped
1C	Cooked macaroni

Sauté garlic and onions in 2 cups water until transparent.

Add celery and carrots.

Continue cooking 5 minutes. Add tomatoes and vegetable broth. Add 2 cups more water to mixture.

Cook 15 minutes, then add remainder of ingredients, except beans and macaroni. Continue to cook 30 minutes on warm, after bringing to a boil. Add beans and simmer on warm for 30 minutes, until done to taste. Add cooked macaroni a few minutes before serving. Makes 8 portions. (1 portion = 215.7 calories, 1.0 grams fat, 19% protein, 77% carbohydrates, 4% fat)

Vegetable Barley Soup

3C	Vegetable broth
2 cans	Tomato sauce
2 large	Carrots, sliced
1 med.	Onion chopped
2 stalks	Celery
1-2	Bay leaves
1 clove	Garlic, chopped
½C	Barley

Combine all ingredients in a large pot.
Bring to a boil, cover, reduce heat and simmer 1 hour. Remove bay leaves and serve. Makes 6 portions. (1 portion = 118.0 calories, 0.7 grams fat, 18% protein, 77% carbohydrates, 5% fat)

Vegetable Entrees

Vegetable Stir Fry

1 can	Mushrooms or ¼ cup dry shiitake mushrooms, soaked and sliced
1 med.	Carrot, sliced diagonally
2 stalks	Broccoli, diagonally sliced
2 stalks	Celery, Diagonally sliced
1½	Round onion, sliced into thin crescents
1 piece	Ginger, crushed
1 clove	Garlic, crushed
1½ Tbsp.	Corn starch
¼C	Water

Seasoning:

1 Tbsp.	Oyster	sauce (vegetarian)
1 tsp.	Soy sauce	
1C	Stock	

Heat pan. Sauté ginger, garlic, and onion in water, remove from pan. Add seasonings and cook 2 minutes. Add stock, mushrooms, carrot, broccoli, and celery and cook until vegetables are crisp and tender. Make a paste with corn starch and water to thicken the gravy. Makes 4 to 6 portions. (1 portion = 59.4 calories, 0.3 grams fat, 19% protein, 77% carbohydrates, 5% fat)

Mu Shu Vegetables

This is a delicious dish that you can get in Szechuan Chinese restaurants by ordering "mu shu pork" but without the pork and eggs.

Mu shu is actually a Chinese delicacy which is a crinkly dark brown fungus. This is difficult to find but not necessary to this dish.
Hoisin sauce, found in the oriental section of the supermarket or in Chinatown, is a savory plum sauce which can make simple vegetables into a feast. It is on the salty and sweet side, so use carefully.

1 pkg.	Mung bean sprouts
1/4 head	Won bok or head cabbage, sliced
1/2	Onion, vertically sliced
4	Shiitake mushrooms, soaked and sliced
1/2	Carrot, julienne
1 clove	Garlic (fresh), minced dash Sesame oil
	Water and soy sauce, to taste
6 tsp.	Hoisin sauce, to taste
6 pieces	Chinese mu shu fungus (optional)
1 bundle	Cellophane noodles, (optional) 1/4 head Cabbage, shredded (optional)
12	Whole wheat chapatis or medium-sized tortillas

Slice cabbage and vertically slice onion into thin crescents. Chop mushrooms and cut carrot into match- sticks or grate it into thin strips.

Soak cellophane noodles in water to cover until soft.

In a large skillet or wok, sauté onions in water and a dash of sesame oil until slightly translucent. Then sauté the rest of the vegetables in water and soy sauce.

Spread 1/2 teaspoon of hoisin sauce on the chapati or tortilla. Lay the sautéed vegetables down the middle. If adding, lay softened cellophane noodles and cabbage on top of vegetables. Roll the vegetables (and noodles) in the chapati or tortilla.

Makes 12 portions.   (1 portion = 145 calories, 2.0 grams fat, 8% protein, 80% carbohydrates, 12% fat)

Vegetable Wraps and Mu Shu Vegetable

Becoming increasingly popular are versatile variations on the vegetable stir fry. Take the leftover stir fry and wrap it in a whole wheat tortilla or chapati (Indian flatbread). For example, you could take leftovers from a stir-fry dinner and in the morning pack a lunch along with some whole wheat tortillas (preferably stone-ground or sprouted grain). Then, at lunch, simply wrap the vegetables in the tortilla - flavor it with soy sauce, barbecue sauce, or any stir-fry sauce of your choice and you have an excellent simple lunch.

As a variation, you can use Hoisin sauce which you can buy where they sell Chinese condiments. This sauce is the secret to a delicious dish usually served at Northern Chinese restaurants called "mushu pork." Of course there is no pork in this dish and it is not necessary. Spreading a thin layer of hoisin sauce makes for a delectable northern Asian dish that you can call "Mushu Vegetable."

Plum Sauce (Hoi Sin Sauce)

Oriental plum sauce is a delicious treat
that can be used for dishes such as "Mu-shu" vegetable. One
variation of plum sauce is known as "Hoisin." You can buy this
bottled, and use it as is. You'll find it in Oriental or health food
stores.

Hawaiian Savory Stew

3 Tbsp.	Water
1 large	Onion, chopped
2 cloves	Garlic, minced
1 piece	Ginger (1"), mashed
1 box	Seitan (wheat gluten), cut in 1" pieces or 1 C mushrooms
1 Tbsp.	Soy sauce
2 large	Carrots, cut in 1" chunks
2 stalks	Celery, cut in 1" chunks
3	Red potatoes, quartered
1 can	Tomatoes, whole packed
3	Bay leaves
2C	Vegetable broth Water, to cover
	Salt, to taste
	Pepper, to taste
2 Tbsp.	Whole wheat flour dissolved in 4 Tbsp. water

Sauté onion and garlic in 3 tablespoons of water in a large pot. Add seitan, ginger, soy sauce, carrots, celery, potatoes, tomatoes, vegetable broth, water to cover, salt, pepper, and bay leaves. Cook until vegetables are tender.   Thicken with whole wheat flour dissolved in 4 tablespoons of water. Serve hot. Zing it with a few drops of Tabasco sauce. Makes 6 to 8 portions. (1 portion = 256.1 calories, 1.2 grams fat, 32% protein, 64% carbohydrates, 4% fat)

Curry Stew

3 Tbsp.	Water
1 lg.	Onion, chopped
2 cloves	Garlic, minced
1 piece	Ginger (1"), mashed
1-2 tsp.	Soy sauce
1 tsp.	Honey
1-3 Tbsp.	Curry powder
2 lg.	Carrots, cut in 1" chunks
2 stalks	Celery, cut in 1" chunks
3	Red potatoes, quartered
3C	Cauliflower florets
½C	Lima beans, frozen
2C	Vegetable broth
	Water, to cover
	Salt, to taste
1 Tbsp.	Corn starch or arrowroot dissolved in 1 tablespoon water

Sauté onion and garlic in 3 tablespoons of water in stainless steel saucepan. Add ginger, soy sauce, honey, curry powder, carrots, celery, potatoes, cauliflower, lima beans, vegetable broth, water to cover, and salt to taste.

Cook for 20 minutes or until carrots become tender. Then thicken with corn starch or arrowroot mixture. Makes 6 portions. (1 portion = 118.5 calories, 0.6 grams fat, 15% protein, 81% carbohydrates, 4% fat)

Mushroom Vegetable Stew

1 med.	Onion, chopped
½ cup	Water
2	Tomatoes, chopped
1 clove	Garlic, minced
3	Carrots, cut into ½" slices
½ lb.	Fresh mushrooms, small
1	small Bell pepper, seeded and diced
3 med.	Red potatoes, unpeeled, cut into ½" cubes
1	Bay leaf
½ tsp.	Basil, dried
½ tsp.	Oregano, diced
½ tsp.	Fine herbs, dried (mixed Italian herbs)
	Salt, to taste
½-1 cup	Green peas, fresh or frozen
1 Tbsp.	Corn starch mixed in 2 Tbsp. water

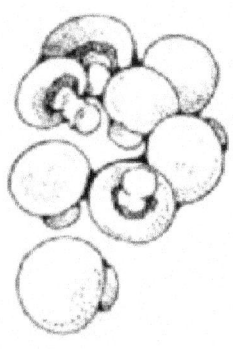

Sauté onions in water until soft. Add other ingredients, holding the salt and peas. Cover and simmer for 30 minutes until vegetables are just tender. Season to taste. Add peas and heat through. Remove bay leaf and thicken with corn starch. Makes 4 portions. (1 portion = 206.4 calories, 0.9 grams fat, 13% protein, 84% carbohydrates, 4% fat)

Cajun Jambalaya

Jambalaya is a Cajun stew.
Cajun cuisine is noted for its hot and spicy bayou flavors. This is a quick, vegetarian version of a favorite bayou dish. If you prefer your foods less spicy, remember that you are always encouraged to adjust these recipes for your own, personal taste.

1 large	Red onion, chopped
1 med.	Yam, peeled and cubed
1	Green bell pepper, chopped
1	Red bell pepper, chopped
1C	Frozen corn
½C	Celery, chopped
1	Bay leaf
3 cloves	Garlic, minced
2 cans	Tomatoes, chopped (with peppers), including liquid (14½ oz.)
1C	Brown rice, precooked
1 tsp.	Dried basil, crushed
1 tsp.	Black pepper
¼ tsp.	Salt
¼ tsp.	Ground red pepper
1 Tbsp.	Tabasco sauce
	Canola oil cooking spray

Spicy Tofu With Cabbagge

16 oz.	Firm tofu
2 lbs.	Won bok, bok choy, or choy sum

Sauce:

1 med.	Onion, minced
2 cloves	Garlic, minced
1C	Vegetable broth
2 tsp.	Red peppers, crushed
2 Tbsp.	Tamari or low-sodium soy sauce
1 tsp.	Sesame oil
1 tsp.	Maple syrup
1 Tbsp.	Corn starch mixed with
2 Tbsp.	water
	Sesame seeds, toasted, to garnish

Drain tofu and cut into squares. Cut cabbage leaves into quarters, then across into 3 sections. Wash, drain, and dry.
Combine sauce ingredients in a large pot and simmer. Thicken with corn starch and water, if desired. Add tofu and keep warm.

Parboil cabbage (adding tougher bottom parts of cabbage first) until crisp-tender. Place cabbage on platter and pour tofu and sauce mixture over. Garnish with sesame seeds and serve.

Makes 6 portions. (1 portion = 170.7 calories, 7.8 grams fat, 35% protein, 26% carbohydrates, 38% fat)

Confetti Rice Stir-Fry

1	Tomato, diced
1	Bell pepper, diced
1 med.	Sweet yellow onion, diced
2	Celery stalks, diced
1C	Snow peas
3 large	Mushrooms, sliced
1 Tbsp.	Vegetable broth powder
	Tamari sauce
2C	Brown rice, cooked
½C	Peas and carrots, frozen
	Canola oil cooking spray

Heat wok to sizzling. Spray lightly with canola oil spray, scald with tamari sauce, toss in vegetables.

When cooked to the desired tenderness, toss with hot brown rice and sunflower seeds. Add a small amount of tamari, to taste. Makes 2 portions. (1 portion = 340.6 calories, 3.2 grams fat, 14% protein, 78% carbohydrates, 8% fat)

Nishime (a form of Japanese stew)

This is a traditional Japanese stew-like dish that is low fat and was one of the favorite dishes on both the HawaiiDiet™ Study and the Program.

2strips	Konbu (dried)
4 pieces	Mushrooms (dried)
2	Konyaku,* sliced
3	Aburage*
1C	Turnip
2C	Japanese taro
1C	Bamboo shoots
1C	Carrots
1C	Burdock root
1 tsp.	Peanut oil
1-1/2 C	Vegetable broth
1/4 C	Tamari
1/3 C	Sugar

 Soak konbu and mushrooms in water until soft, about 10 minutes.

Wash and scrub Japanese taro thoroughly until clean. Peel and cut into 1-1/2" pieces.

Cut konbu, konyaku, aburage, turnip, bamboo shoots, and carrots into 1-1/2" pieces. Cut burdock root into 1/4"-thick diagonal slices and soak in water until used.

Tie konbu into knots leaving 1" apart. Cut between knots.

In a saucepan, add peanut oil, vegetable broth, mush-rooms, konbu, konyaku, and bamboo shoots. Cover and cook for 10 minutes. Add tamari and sugar; cook for 5 minutes. Add turnip, carrots, and burdock root and cook for 15 minutes. Add taro and cook until taro is fork tender.

Toss in aburage and serve.

Makes 4 portions. Taro must be cooked properly. Do NOT eat raw.

* Konnyaku is a chewy product made from yam flour. Aburage is fried tofu skin, also used for cone sushi. Both are available where Japanese foods are sold.

Monk's Food

This Peace Diet recipe section wouldn't be complete without an example of a recipe for Chinese "monk's food" or "Jai". It is the quintessential dish that represents the ancient belief that vegetarian food helps to nurture the spirit. It has remained in Chinese tradition prominently enough that most Chinese restaurants will serve "Jai" or "Chai" at Chinese New Year because it is supposed to be a dish that helps to cleanse the soul. It is always purely vegan with an assortment of exotic vegetables and other non-animal ingredients. They usually have 10 or more ingredients, some of them quite exotic and difficult to find such as "wood ear" or black fungus, lotus seeds, and lily flowers. If you can find these items, please add them, but this is a recipe with ingredients that are easier to find.

Lo Han Jai (Lo Han means "enlightened person" Jai means vegetarian dish)

6-8 oz	Long rice, thin diameter,
5 pieces,	Shitake Mushroom, soaked & quartered
1/2 pkg or 6 oz,	Flavored or plain firm tofu, cubed
1/2 inch thick piece,	Ginger, thinly sliced
2-3 C	Won Bok or Chinese Cabbage, cut into thick vertical slices
1/2,	Carrot, thinly sliced
½ C,	Snow peas, whole or halved
½ C*	Canned water chestnuts,
1-2 tsp	Tamari soy sauce (or any light to medium colored soy sauce),
2 Tbsp	Vegetarian Mushroom Sauce, or 2 tsp Better Than Bouillion Veggie Base,

94

½ C	Water to dilute mushroom sauce or veggie base,
1 Tbsp	Cornstarch,
	Water to mix in corn starch,
1 C	Maple syrup
1 t	Sea salt, 2 t or to taste
	Chili flakes, a big pinch (optional)
2 T	Cooking oil

Cut long rice in half and soak in water for ten minutes. Boil in hot water until softened. Drain and set aside. Soak shitake mushroom until pliable and cut each piece into quarters. Squeeze out water. Heat wok or frying pan with 2 t of oil and sautee ginger and mushrooms in medium low heat. Add ½ C of water or more if necessary and cook until mushrooms are tender. Remove from pan.

Fry Tofu cubes in 1 t of oil in medium low heat until golden brown. Remove from pan.

Fry carrots in remaining oil in high heat for 2-3 minutes before adding remaining vegetables. Cook for 3 more minutes. Reduce heat to medium low and add in tofu, sautéed mushrooms and long rice. Combine well and cook for a few more minutes.
Stir in seasoning and pour in cornstarch and water mixture and cook for 2-3 minutes in low heat. Add more water if necessary to ensure perfect consistency. Allow long rice to absorb all or most of the liquid. Remove from wok and serve immediately. Serves 2-3.

Notes: Water chestnuts can be substituted with cooked lotus seeds or roasted peanuts. Cooking oil for frying can be substituted with water or vegetable broth. Provided Courtesy of OriAnn Li, Author, Vegan Paradise, www.oriannli.com

Zucchini Caliente

Caliente means "fiery." The key to this dish is to make it just hot enough, without being too hot. If you like mild dishes, you'll want to cut down on the spices here. If you like your food hot, leave as is and serve with a side dish of jalapeños.

2 tsp.	Olive oil
1C	Onions, chopped
1C	Sweet red pepper, chopped
2 cloves	Garlic, finely chopped
2½ C	Zucchini, unpeeled, cut into ¼" slices
1 lb.	Tomatoes, chopped
¼C	Tomato juice
¼ tsp.	Coriander, ground
½ tsp.	Cumin, ground
½ tsp.	Chili powder
	Salt to taste

Sauté onions, pepper, and garlic in a large nonstick skillet, until tender, about 10 minutes. Add zucchini, tomatoes, and tomato juice. Sprinkle spices evenly over vegetables. Mix well. Cover and cook 5 minutes, until zucchini is tender-crisp. Makes 4 portions. (1 portion = 91.4 calories, 3.0 grams fat,   13% protein, 62% carbohydrates, 26% fat)

Vegetable Side Dishes

Vegetable side dishes should be an important part of your Peace Diet. Steamed vegetables are easy to prepare and are a versatile way to add taste, healthfulness and color to your meal. There are several techniques for steaming, including a bamboo basket over boiling water, a metal steamer over boiling water, or a modern electric steamer that is compact, low cost, has a timer, and makes your steaming foolproof.   Vegetables can also be baked or sautéed depending on the type of vegetable. Whatever form your vegetables take, they are surprisingly rich in nutrients. Here's some information about a few vegetables; it's fairly representative of the nutrient value of vegetables in general:

- Cauliflower – This cruciferous vegetable, popular for the way it blends and enhances the food it is cooked with, is very high in vitamin C but extremely low in calories and has no fat.
- Broccoli – Another cruciferous vegetable, broccoli is so versatile it can be used in salads, side dishes, soups, stir-frys, or dips. It enhances the other ingredients it is served with, while providing vitamin A, C, calcium, fiber, phytonutrients, and very low calories.
- Carrots – This vegetable may be taken for granted, but it is packed with vitamin A (betacarotene), which is so good for the eyes. Its soluble fiber is good for cholesterol as well.

Some steamed vegetables such as cauliflower, broccoli, julienned carrots, zucchini squash, and so on, are especially good with dipping sauces. These same vegetables may be sliced and used raw, too. Use the sauces above to dip them in, experiment with a variety of them. You'll find that turning your vegetable dishes into wholesome easy snacks - whether raw or steamed - is one of the easiest ways for you to get your several servings of vegetables per day. Try sauces to give your vegetables variety. You'll find several sauces in the Kebob section (p. 173) of these recipes. You can also try the salad dressings for dips as well.

Vegetable Kebobs

Here's an experiment for you. Try taking a piece of meat and chewing it about 100 times. You will for the first time learn the true taste of meat. It tastes like cardboard or worse.

Kebobs taste good because of the sauce, so you don't need the meat. The trick is to get the right sauce. One was so good that one of my patients took vegetable kebobs to a party, used the Dijon marinade and found that even the meat eaters enjoyed them. In fact, they liked the dish so much, they were taking the meat off their kebobs, using my friend's sauce, and enjoying a better tasting kebob.

Simple Vegetable Kebob:

• Try vegetable kebobs with vegetables of your choice such as broccoli, mushrooms, zucchini, onions, cauliflower, bell peppers, or carrots. Cut them into chunks and place them on skewers. Marinate thoroughly with your favorite marinade sauce. Then, roast over an open fire or grill.

• Use one of the sauces below. Personally, my favorite is the Dijon Sauce.

Sauces and Gravies

Sauces and gravies enhance the flavor of your meals. Unfortunately, most of the sauces and gravies we grew up eating were made from a base of animal grease and/or cream, both high in fat. With the following recipes, the Eat More, Weigh Less™ Diet once again proves that low fat doesn't have to mean low taste. You can eat gravy again. Just learn the Eat More, Weigh Less™ Tips and stick to the low-fat recipes below. Use these gravies and sauces to dress up vegetables, beans, noodles or grains. Mix and match, use your creativity. You'll soon be turning simple dishes into something special.

Sauces For Steamed Vegetables

Steamed vegetables should be a staple part of your Eat More, Weigh Less™ Diet. There are several techniques for steaming, including a bamboo basket over boiling water, a metal steamer over boiling water, or a modern electric steamer that is compact, low   cost (between $20-$30), has a timer, and makes your steaming foolproof. If at all possible, invest in an electric steamer. A good one is a Black and Decker®, at about $30. It will make your steaming so simple that you'll do a whole lot more of it, and steaming is one of the healthiest ways to prepare your food. A good combination of steamed vegetables, for use with dipping sauces, is cauliflower, broccoli, julienned carrots, zucchini squash, and so on. These same vegetables may be sliced and used raw, too. Use the sauces above to dip them in, experiment with a variety of them. You'll find that turning your vegetable dishes into wholesome easy snacks - whether raw or steamed - is one of the easiest ways for you to get your 3 to 5 servings of vegetables per day. Try sauces to give your vegetables variety.

Dijon Mustard Sauce

One of my favorite sauces is what I call "3221" sauce. This is a lip-smacking mustard sauce that can be used to make vegetables absolutely delicious. It's also simple to prepare.

It's called "3221" because you use:

3 Tbsp.	Dijon mustard
2 Tbsp.	Soy sauce
2 Tbsp.	Lemon juice or balsamic vinegar
1 clove	Garlic, crushed

Mix them all togjether, and you have a delicious dipping sauce that is out of this world. It's incredibly easy. Try it and see. Makes 3 portions. (1 portion = 25.6 calories, 0.6 grams fat, 26% protein, 52% carbohydrates, 22% fat)

Asian Sauce

Oriental sauce is delicious on vegetables.

You can make a variety of these sauces from scratch, or buy them bottled. Also, for your convenience, you can use a vegetarian oyster sauce, a miso sauce, or a ginger sauce. Ginger is a superb condiment and can be used as an ingredient in any number of different sauces. Ginger has a little bit of zip, similar to horseradish or chili sauce.

Oriental Ginger Sauce

1C	Water
4 Tbsp.	Low-sodium soy sauce
1 Tbsp.	Arrowroot or corn starch
1 Tbsp.	Ginger, grated

Mix arrowroot or corn starch in ¼ cup of cool water. Add to a saucepan with the water, soy sauce, and ginger. Heat at medium until thickened and stir.

Serve with steamed vegetables. Makes 10 portions. (1 portion = 6.9 calories, 0.0 grams   fat,   21%   protein,   78% carbohydrates, 1% fat)

Miso-Based Sauce

Miso-based sauces are also savory on vegetables. All you have to do is dilute some miso with a little bit of flour, water and other spices, then use this as a delicious dipping sauce for raw or steamed vegetables. You can also use this sauce as a variation when you're making a stir-fry.

Ginger Miso Sauce

4 Tbsp.	Sweet white miso
1 Tbsp.	Fresh ginger juice
1 Tbsp.	Ginger, grated
1 clove	Garlic (large), minced
	Juice of one lemon
½ tsp.	Corn starch (for thicker sauce)
1C	Water

Blend ingredients until well mixed, then heat gently. Add corn starch for a thicker sauce. Serve over vegetables, use as dipping sauce, or use as base in stir-frys. Keeps well. Makes 8 portions. (1 portion = 22.7 calories, 0.6 grams fat, 19% protein, 59% carbohydrates, 21% fat)

Curry Sauce

Curry sauce is an exotic dipping sauce you can use to impress your friends - or to treat yourself. Because the ingredient list is long, most people think it will be difficult to prepare. However, once you have the ingredients together, the sauce can be deceptively simple to make. Try the following recipe on vegetables, seitan, tempeh, and other meat substitutes; in corn dishes or over whole grains.

Simple Curry Sauce

4 tsp.	Whole wheat flour
2 tsp.	Curry powder (choose mild, medium or hot, to taste)
1C	Vegetable broth
1C	Water
2 tsp.	Ginger, finely chopped
1 med.	Onion, chopped
1	Bay leaf
1 clove	Garlic, crushed

Blend all ingredients, then cook over medium heat until thickened.   Simmer 10 minutes. Remove bay leaf. Makes 24 portions. (1 portion = 6.2 calories, 0.1 grams fat, 19% protein, 74% carbohydrates, 7% fat)

Barbecue Sauce

Barbecue sauces are great for dressing up vegetables. They also make good sauces for sandwich fillings and protein-based foods such as the meat substitutes.

You can make your own sauce, or barbecue sauce can be bought in the store. Most of these sauces are low in fat. Nevertheless, make sure that you read the bottle or you might be surprised.

The brands of bottled barbecue sauces I recommend include the following: Robbie's Barbecue Sauce®, Hickory Flavor; Bull's Eye Original Barbecue Sauce®; and Hunt's All Natural Thick & Rich Barbecue Sauce®, to name a few.

BBQ Sauce

½C	Water
1 tsp.	Soy sauce
1 large	Onion, minced
3 cloves	Garlic, minced
1 can	Tomato sauce (8 oz.)
1C	Tomato ketchup
1C	Water
1 Tbsp.	Honey
1 tsp.	Chili powder
2 Tbsp.	Cider vinegar
1 tsp.	Dry mustard
2 Tbsp.	Tamari
½ Tbsp.	Corn starch, whole wheat flour, dissolved
in	2 tablespoons water

In a large pan, heat water and soy sauce.

Add chopped onion and the garlic. Cook until the onion is soft. Add other ingredients and cook over medium heat for 10 minutes. Stir often.

To thicken, add corn starch, whole wheat flour, or kuzu, dissolved in water. Makes 36 portions. (1 portion = 22.8 calories, 0.1 grams fat, 10% protein, 85% carbohydrates, 5% fat)

Tofu Sauce

Some people like creamy sauces. Tofu provides a creamy texture for vegetables dips and other dishes, and is somewhat similar in texture to mayonnaise, a dish that most of us grew up with. A lot of people like mayonnaise but don't want the high-fat content. (Mayonnaise is almost totally fat, at about 12 grams of fat per tablespoon, and with about 98% of its calories coming from fat.)

Tofu-based sauces are far better than that.

But don't forget, tofu still has a fair amount of fat. It's 51% fat by calories, with about 5 grams of fat per quarter pound. It has about 0.8 grams of fat per tablespoon. This means it's not all that good for you when you're watching your weight. But it's still a lot better than the 12 grams of fat per tablespoon in regular mayonnaise.

Using tofu as a sauce base saves you about 11 grams of fat per tablespoon. That's not bad. In addition, tofu is moderate on the EMI scale, whereas mayonnaise is at rock bottom. To use tofu as a sauce base, put it in a blender with a couple of other ingredients and blend until smooth. Try the following recipe for tofu mayonnaise, use it on sandwiches, vegetables, and other places where you might ordinarily use mayonnaise.

Tofu Dip Sauce

1 blk.	Soft tofu (16 oz.)
1 Tbsp.	Onion, minced
½C	Vegetarian broth (e.g., vegetarian chicken, konbu, etc.)
2 Tbsp.	Low-sodium soy sauce (or to taste)
1 tsp.	Lemon juice

Mash tofu and mix in other ingredients.

Place in a blender and puree. Use this as a vegetable topping or a dip for steamed vegetables. Makes 20 portions. (1 portion = 14.2 calories, 0.6 grams fat, 34% protein,   26% carbohydrates, 40% fat)

Mediterranean Herb Sauce

Mediterranean dishes are characterized by the creative use of herbs, spices, vinegar, olive oil, and even wine. The trick to making use of these flavors in the Eat More, Weigh Less™ Diet is to eliminate or minimize the olive oil. As good as olive oil may be in other respects, in terms of weight loss, it has the same number of calories (9 calories per gram), the same low EMI value, and the same potential for making weight loss difficult as do other fats and oils. So concentrate on the delicious other flavors such as basil, garlic, oregano, etc., and be creative with Mediterranean sauces for pastas and vegetables.

1 clove	Garlic, minced
2 Tbsp.	Dijon mustard
½C	Red wine vinegar
1 tsp.	Black pepper
½C	Basil leaves, sliced
½ tsp.	Onion powder
1 Tbsp.	Honey

Combine all ingredients and serve over steamed vegetables. Could be used as a marinade or over vegetable kebobs. Makes 7 portions. (1 portion = 17.1 calories, 0.3 grams fat, 8% protein, 80% carbohydrates, 12% fat)

Steamed Garlic Broccoli

This is a simple, high-calcium dish that can be used as a side dish to just about any entrée. In addition to being high in calcium, broccoli is a "cruciferous vegetable," which means it is loaded with anti-cancer nutrients such as beta carotene, indole amines, and fiber. Steamed Garlic Broccoli was served on the Hawaii Health Program as well as the Hawaii-Diet™ Study.

1 bunch	Broccoli, chopped
1 clove	Garlic, minced
1/2 C	Water
	sprinkle Sesame seed, roasted or sesame salt

Wash and chop the broccoli, separating the stems and flowerettes. Place the broccoli stems in a 1-1/2- quart saucepan with the water and garlic; cover and steam for 4 minutes. Uncover and stir the stems, arrange the flowerettes on top, then cover and steam for another 4 minutes.

Serve with a sprinkling of roasted sesame seeds or sesame salt (gomasio). Makes 4 portions. (1 portion = 28 calories, 0.3 gram fat, 33% protein, 59% carbohydrates, 8% fat)

Melt-In-Your-Mouth Kabocha Squash

1 Kabocha or acorn squash

Cut the kabocha squash into 4" squares or cleaned acorn squash in quarters. Place on a baking pan with a tiny bit of water and bake at 350degrees F. until tender (about an hour). Makes 2 portions. (1 portion = 115.0 calories, 0.290 grams fat, 7% protein, 91% carbohydrates, 2% fat)

For a little zing, try adding a tablespoon of miso and a teaspoon of sweetener such as barley malt. (See Squash Deluxe in the Eat More, Weigh Less™ Diet Book, page 215.)

▽ Remember, you can eat the skin and all, so
wash it all before you prepare it. For a more elaborate
squash dish, try the following recipe.   ▽

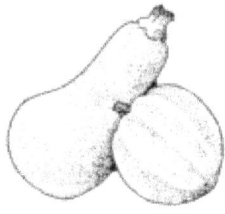

Butternut Squash with Whole Wheat, Wild Rice, and Onion Stuffing

This satisfying dish makes an especially handsome centerpiece for a holiday meal such as Thanksgiving.

4	Butternut squashes (medium-small, about 1 lb. each)
2C	Water
	Canola oil cooking spray
1C	Red onion (heaping), chopped
1 clove	Garlic, minced
1C	Fresh orange juice
2½ C	Whole wheat bread, torn and firmly packed
¾C	Wild rice, raw, rinsed
½ tsp.	Dried sage
½ tsp.	Dried thyme

In the meantime, bring the water to a boil in a saucepan. Stir in the wild rice, reduce to a simmer, then cover and cook until the water is absorbed, about 40 minutes.

Spray heating skillet with canola oil cooking spray. Add the onion and garlic and sauté until the onion is limp and golden.

113

In a mixing bowl, combine the cooked wild rice with the sautéed onion and the remaining ingredients. When the squashes are cool enough to handle, scoop out the pulp, leaving firm shells about ½" thick. Chop the pulp and stir it into the rice mixture. Stuff the squashes, place in foil-lined baking dishes, and cover.

Before oserving, place the squashes in a preheated 350 F. Bake for 20 minutes, or until well heated through. Makes 8 portions. (1 portion = 259.9 calories, 2.2 grams fat, 12% protein, 81% carbohydrates, 7% fat)

Broccoli With Mustard Sauce

This is another simple, high-calcium dish.

1 bunch	Broccoli
1/2 cup	Rice vinegar (seasoned)
2 tsp.	Mustard (Stone ground or Dijon-style)
1-2 cloves	Garlic, pressed or minced

Break broccoli into bite-sized flowerettes. Peel the stems and slice them into 1/4" thick rounds. Steam until just tender, about 3 minutes. While broccoli is steaming, whisk the remaining ingredients in a serving bowl. Add the steamed broccoli and toss to mix. Serve immediately.

Makes 4 portions.   (1 portion = 36 calories, 0.4 gram fat, 28% protein, 64% carbohydrates, 8% fat)

Baked Eggplant Marinara

1½ lbs.	Eggplant, unpeeled, cut into 12 slices
14 oz.	Low-fat spaghetti sauce
	Olive oil cooking spray

Coat baking sheet with olive oil cooking spray. Add sliced eggplant, put about 1 tablespoon of spaghetti sauce on each slice, spread to cover.

Bake at 350 degrees Farenheit. oven for about 30 to 35 minutes. Eggplant slices are done when they are tender enough to be easily pierced with a fork. Serve in sandwiches, as a side dish, or in other creative ways. Makes 4 portions.

Wakame with Mixed Vegetables

Wakame with mixed vegetables is another high calcium dish primarily because of the seaweed (wakame).

2-1/2 oz.	Wakame, dried
5C	Daikon, sliced
5C	Carrots, sliced
5C	Cauliflower, cut
5C	Turnips, sliced
8 Tbsp.	Soy sauce (low sodium)
	Water
	Green onions (garnish)

Rinse and soak wakame. Slice into large pieces.
Put other vegetables in a large soup pot and half cover with water. Bring to a boil, cover, and reduce heat to low, simmering until the vegetables are almost cooked. Add wakame and low-sodium soy sauce to taste until the vegetables are cooked. Serve one cup in a bowl and garnish with green onions.

Makes 20 portions. (1 portion = 47 calories, 0.3 grams fat, 17% protein, 78% carbohydrates, 5% fat)

Mock Crabmeat Sauce Over Broccoli

This was very highly rated by the participants on the HawaiiDiet™ Study and on the Hawaii Health Program.

1-1/2 lb.	Broccoli
1 cake	Tofu
1 tsp.	Sesame oil
1 tsp.	Peanut oil
1-1/2 tsp.	Garlic, minced
2 tsp.	Ginger (fresh), minced
5 Tbsp.	White table wine
2 tsp.	Salt
1/2 C	Water Sugar
1/4 tsp.	White pepper, freshly ground
2	Egg whites, beaten
1-1/2	Cornstarch, mixed with 1 Tbsp. water
3 Tbsp.	Carrot, minced

Wash and cut broccoli flowerettes and stems. Cut stems in 1" diagonal pieces. Steam broccoli in steamer for 3 minutes. Mash tofu with fork and add 1/2 teaspoon sesame oil. Heat wok or skillet to high and add peanut oil. Add garlic and ginger and cook for 10 seconds. Add broccoli, 3-1/2 tablespoons of wine, 1-1/2 teaspoon salt, sesame oil and stir fry for 1 minute. Remove and set on platter. Clean the wok or skillet. Reheat wok to high and add mashed tofu and stir fry for 30 seconds. Add 1/2 cup of water, 1-1/2 tablespoons wine, 1/2 teaspoon salt, 1/2 teaspoon sugar, 1/4 teaspoon pepper and 2 beaten egg whites. Cook for 20 seconds. Slowly add cornstarch mixture, stirring constantly until sauce thickens. Pour mixture over broccoli and sprinkle minced carrot over broccoli. Serve immediately. Makes 4 portions. (1 portion = 120 calories, 4.1 grams fat, 30% protein, 40% carbohydrates, 30% fat)

Broccoli With Mustard Sauce

This is another simple, high-calcium dish.

1 bunch	Broccoli
1/2 cup	Rice vinegar (seasoned)
2 tsp.	Mustard (Stone ground or Dijon-style)
1-2 cloves	Garlic, pressed or minced

Break broccoli into bite-sized flowerettes. Peel the stems and slice them into 1/4" thick rounds. Steam until just tender, about 3 minutes. While broccoli is steaming, whisk the remaining ingredients in a serving bowl. Add the steamed broccoli and toss to mix. Serve immediately.

Makes 4 portions.   (1 portion = 36 calories, 0.4 gram fat, 28% protein, 64% carbohydrates, 8% fat)

High Calcium Vegetables

Many people have been raised on dairy, so they automatically see that as the natural source for calcium. They don't realize that vegetables are actually the best source of calcium. Think for a minute. After all, where do cows get calcium? They don't eat dairy. They eat greens. And if you are concerned about osteoporosis, remember that the countries that consume the most dairy have the most osteoporosis in their population. So where do we get calcium?

Fortunately, nature provides plenty of calcium in dark leafy greens and sea vegetables. Steam or par-boil them and if you wish, flavor them with one of the sauces described in this book for kebobs. Here are some examples that you can use as high calcium side dishes.

- Broccoli is one of the best sources of calcium. One-half cup daily exceeds the recommended daily allowance (RDA) of both vitamin C and E.
- Kale contains more calcium than milk, ounce for ounce. Its calcium is more absorbable by the body than milk. Its calcium protects against osteoporosis, arthritis, and bone loss.
- Collard greens include not only calcium but also the key ingredients of iron, magnesium, potassium, sodium, zinc, copper, manganese, vitamin C, B, E, and several phytochemicals.

- Watercress is an excellent source of calcium and antioxidants for fighting cancer, but also treats anemia, calcium deficiencies, liver and pancreatic problems, thyroid problems, and arthritis.
- Beet or turnip greens provide calcium, minerals, and carotenes. They provide vitamins and phytochemicals.
- Bok choy is an excellent source of highly absorbable calcium as well as beta-carotene to battle heart disease and cancer.
- Mustard cabbage (napa cabbage) also contains highly absorbable calcium and iron. It protects against cancer and heart disease and strengthens the immune system.

Other good sources of calcium are wakame and kelp (sea vegetables, see below).   Don't forget that there is also a fair amount of calcium in beans as well.

Taking a calcium supplement with magnesium and vitamin D is another option if you are sure you won't be eating greens.

Zesty Broccoli

1 bunch	Broccoli
1	Lemon or lemon juice
2 tsp	Garlic powder
	Soy sauce to taste

Wash the broccoli and peel off the fibrous part of the stem. Then cut into bite-sized flowerets. Steam or par-boil until barely fork-tender and still bright green. Drain the water and then, squeeze lemon juice onto each floweret. Then sprinkle the garlic powder and a little soy sauce or Bragg's liquid aminos to taste. (Hint: if you have a Bragg's liquid amino spray bottle, it is easier to distribute the soy sauce or liquid aminos evenly).

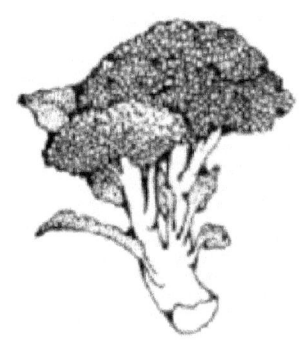

Sea Vegetables

Sea vegetables come in many varieties. We associate them with Japan and China, but really they are collected from all over the world. It is marine algae which grows in shallow waters on ocean shores.

These exotic vegetables supply our greatest source of minerals and trace elements. They contain alginic acid which has the ability to detoxify the body by binding with any heavy metals and causing them to be released from our bodies. Sea vegetables are also high in protein and fiber, with significant amounts of calcium, iron, potassium, phosphorus, magnesium, zinc, iodine, and vitamins A, C, E, K, and B-complex.

Probably the easiest way to use seaweed is to add it to soup. You can add wakame to any soup you can think of and it will add an excellent source of minerals and flavor. Soup recipes are in the section following these seaweed side dishes.

Watercress Sesame Salad

1 bunch	Watercress, cut into
1½"	lengths
2C	Water, boiling
2 Tbsp.	Low-sodium soy sauce
1½ Tbsp.	Sesame seed, toasted
2 Tbsp.	Rice wine vinegar
2 Tbsp.	Green onions including stems, chopped
¼ tsp.	Cayenne
1 clove	Garlic, minced
¼ tsp.	Honey

Place watercress in boiling water and cook for about 4 minutes, rinse and drain thoroughly. Add remaining ingredients and mix well. Chill before serving. Makes 4 portions. (1 portion = 32.3 calories, 1.6 grams fat, 18% protein, 42% carbohydrates, 41% fat)

Here's another excellent high-calcium dish.

Spicy Broccoli

1 bunch	Broccoli
2 tsp.	Dry mustard
½C	Seasoned rice vinegar
2 cloves	Garlic, pressed or minced
¼C	Onion, minced
2 Tbsp.	Honey
2 Tbsp.	Low-sodium soy sauce

Break broccoli into bite- sized florets. Slice peeled stems into ¼" thick rounds. Steam until tender (about 3 minutes).

While broccoli is steaming, mix other ingredients in a serving bowl.   Add broccoli and mix.

Serve immediately. Makes 4 portions. (1 portion = 68.1 calories, 0.6 grams fat, 16% protein, 77% carbohydrates, 7% fat)

Wakame with Mixed Vegetables

Wakame with mixed vegetables is another high calcium dish primarily because of the seaweed (wakame).

2-1/2 oz. Wakame, dried Daikon, sliced
5C Carrots, sliced
5C Cauliflower, cut Turnips, sliced
5C Soy sauce (low sodium)
5C Water
8 Tbsp. Green onions (garnish)

Rinse and soak wakame. Slice into large pieces.
Put other vegetables in a large soup pot and half

cover with water. Bring to a boil, cover, and reduce heat to low, simmering until the vegetables are almost cooked. Add wakame and low-sodium soy sauce to taste until the vegetables are cooked. Serve one cup in a bowl and garnish with green onions. Makes 20 portions. (1 portion = 47 calories, 0.3 grams fat, 17% protein, 78% carbohydrates, 5% fat)

Wakame with Carrots

Wakame with carrots is a variation on the previous recipe that is not only high in calcium but also in beta carotene and the family of carotenoids which are powerful antioxidants.

2 oz.	Wakame (dried)
4C	Carrots, cut into large chunks
	Water to cover vegetables
2 Tbsp.	Soy sauce (low sodium)
	Cilantro, scallions, or parsley (garnish)

Rinse and soak wakame. Slice into large pieces.
Put the carrots in a pot and add water to half cover the carrots. Bring to a boil, cover, and reduce heat to low. Simmer until the carrots are nearly cooked, about 20 to 30 minutes. Then add the soy sauce and wakame. Simmer until carrots are done. Garnish.

Makes 4 portions.   (1 portion = 60 calories, 0.3 gram fat, 14% protein, 82% carbohydrates, 4% fat)

Wakame Namasu

"Namasu" is a traditional Japanese dish which literally means "raw with vinegar," so this is a dish of raw vegetables with a sweet vinegar dressing. You can actually use this preparation with just about any raw vegetables for a great, tasty, no-fat meal. Wakame, which is a tender, leafy sea vegetable, lends itself well with this dish and is also high in calcium.

1/4 C	Vinegar
3 Tbsp.	Honey
1/2 tsp.	Salt
1/2 tsp.	Ginger (fresh), grated
	Juice from 1/2 lemon or lime
1 pkg.	Wakame (1 oz.)
1	Carrot

Combine vinegar, honey, salt, ginger, and lemon or lime juice. Set aside.

Julienne carrot and sprinkle with salt. Let stand for about 30 minutes. Rinse and squeeze water from carrots. Soak wakame in cold water just until hydrated. Squeeze out excess water. Combine wakame, carrots, and sauce. Serve.

Makes 4 portions. (1 portion = 64 calories, 0.1 gram fat, 3% protein, 96% carbohydrates, 1% fat)

Ginger Mustard Cabbage with Konbu

Mustard cabbage and konbu (seaweed) are both excellent sources of calcium and this is a versatile side dish to complement most entrées.

2 lbs.	Mustard cabbage
1 Tbsp.	Sea salt
1/3 C	Konbu (dried), cut in 1/2" strips
1/3 C	Barley malt
1/4 C	Soy sauce (low sodium)
1/4 C	Rice vinegar
1 Tbsp.	Sesame seeds, toasted
1 Tbsp.	Ginger root, minced

Chop cabbage, add salt, and let stand for 30 minutes. Wash konbu and soak until soft. Drain and discard liquid, then cut into 1/2" lengths.

In a saucepan, mix barley malt and soy sauce. Heat until sugar dissolves. Add vinegar then konbu while still hot. Cool the sauce a little, then mix in the rest of ingredients. Transfer to a storage container and let sit over- night in refrigerator to blend flavors.

Makes four (8-ounce) portions.   (1 serving = 85 calories, 1.6 grams fat, 15% protein, 75% carbohydrates, 10% fat)

Vegetable Staples

Roasted Potatoes

This dish brings out the full flavor of potatoes and yet limits the fat to under 2 grams and less than 10% of calories as compared to typical fried potatoes (which would be about 8 grams of fat and 48% fat by calories per serving).

1-1/2 lb.	Red potatoes, unpeeled
1 head	Garlic, roasted
1/4 C	Rosemary, chopped
	Salt, to taste
	Black pepper, freshly ground, to taste
	Olive oil cooking spray

Preheat oven to 375° F.
Cut potatoes in halves and place in baking pan. Cut ends of garlic and spread over roasted potatoes. Spray olive oil and sprinkle with rosemary. Cover pan and bake for 20 minutes. Remove cover and roast for 10 to 15 minutes. Season with salt and pepper.

Makes 3 portions.   (1 portion = 273 calories, 1.2 grams fat, 9% protein, 87% carbohydrates, 4% fat)

Teriyaki Potatoes

For a change of pace in potatoes, try this East-West variation that combines great tastes of two worlds - baked potatoes with "teriyaki" taste.

1/2 C	Soy sauce
3 Tbsp.	Brown sugar
3 cloves	Garlic, mashed
1 piece	Ginger, 1", mashed
2 stalks	Green onion, chopped
1 tsp.	Sesame oil
	Black pepper, to taste
	Red potatoes, peeled and quartered

Preheat oven to 375° F.

In a bowl combine soy sauce, brown sugar, garlic, ginger, green onion, sesame oil, and black pepper; mix well.

Place the potatoes in this same bowl and marinate overnight, stirring occasionally.

Line a baking pan with aluminum foil and place the marinated potatoes in the middle of the pan.

Bake for 25 to 30 minutes, basting with the marinade. Broil the potatoes the last 10 minutes for a crispy texture.

Makes 8 portions.   (1 portion = 136 calories, 0.7 gram fat, 10% protein, 85% carbohydrates, 5% fat)

Chestnut Stuffing

Great for holidays or anytime that you want an alternative to mashed potatoes or other starchy staples.

1/2 C	Onion, minced
1-2 stalks	Celery
1	Apple, minced
8-10	Water chestnuts, chopped
1 tsp.	Salt
1 tsp.	Sage
1 tsp.	Thyme
1/2 tsp.	Pepper
5C	Whole wheat bread and white bread, cubed and mixed together
1/2 lb.	Chestnuts, boiled (breadfruit, in season, can be used)
3/4 C	Chicken-flavored broth

Water-sauté onions, celery, apple, and water chest-nuts. When onions are translucent add salt, sage, thyme, and pepper. Add bread cubes and chestnuts, alternating with chicken flavored broth.

Makes 10 portions. (1 portion = 179 calories, 2.3 grams fat, 12% protein, 77% carbohydrates, 11% fat)

Steamed Sweet Potatoes or Yams

6 med.   Sweet potatoes or yams
                               Water

Place whole sweet potatoes in steamer with 1" of water and steam for approximately 15 minutes or until fork tender. Slice and serve. Or create glazed sweet potatoes by covering with the following sauce and baking for 5 more minutes. Makes 6 portions. (1 sweet potato portion = 117.0 calories, 0.125 grams fat, 7% protein, 93% carbohydrates, 1% fat) (1 yam portion = 127.8 calories, 0.1 grams fat, 5% protein, 94% carbohydrates, 1% fat)

Sweet potatoes and yams are simple and simply delicious by themselves. They are great at any meal or as snacks.

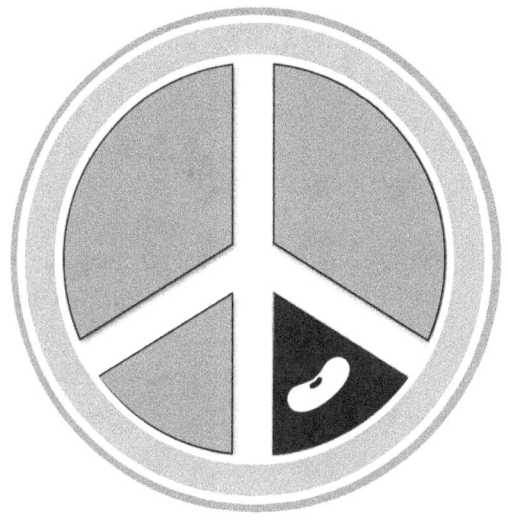

Beans and Legumes

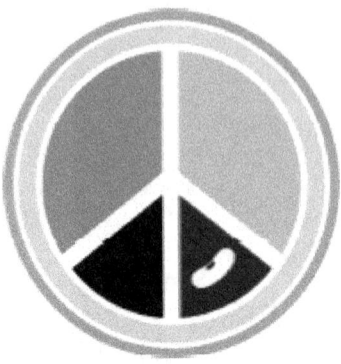

BEANS

Beans are delicious, hearty and filling and a great source of protein and iron. They can be calorically dense, but they can be excellent weight loss dishes when prepared properly. Moderate to high on the SMI, they make delicious dips and spreads that are very low in fat (as long as you don't add any fats).

From a health standpoint, beans are not only fat free but research associates them with lower rates of heart disease and some cancers. Beans provide significant amounts of folate, manganese, magnesium, copper, iron, and potassium – nutrients we don't always get enough of.

Beans come in a variety of shapes, colors, and sizes, which add interest to cooking and eating. Dried beans are the least expensive, but take longer to prepare. They last for a year or more in an airtight container.

If you don't have time to cook, pick up a can at the supermarket or the health food store. Simply drain and use these beans as if they were cooked beans.

Regular Pot			Pressure Cooker	
1 cup of beans	cups of water	time	cups of water	time
Lentils	3	30-60 min.	to cover	10-20 min.
Split Peas	3-Feb	30-60 min.	1/2" over	10 min.
Black Beans	4	1.5-2 hrs.	3/4" over	10-20 min.
Kidney Beans	3	1.5-2 hrs.	1/2" over	15-20 min.
Navy Beans	2	1.5-2 hrs.	1/2" over	10-20 min.
Pinto Beans	3	2-2.5 hrs.	1/2" over	10-20 min.
Chickpeas (garbanos)	2	2.5-3 hrs.	1/2" over	15-25 min.
Azuki Beans	3	2-2.5 hrs.	1/2" over	15-20 min.
Soy Beans	4-Mar	3-4 hrs	3/4" over	30 min.

Chunky Three-Bean Chili

3 large	Sweet onions, diced
2C	Plum tomatoes, chopped
4 cloves	Garlic, minced
1 tsp.	Ground cumin
6C	Vegetable broth (or more, as needed)
2 Tbsp.	Chili powder or to taste
1C	Garbanzo beans, soaked and drained
1C	Kidney beans, soaked and drained
1C	Pinto beans, soaked and drained
¼C	Green chilies, canned and diced
3 Tbsp.	Low-sodium tomato paste
1 tsp.	Dried basil
	Olive oil cooking spray

Spray large pot with cooking spray. Heat 3 tablespoons vegetable broth and sauté onions, garlic, and cumin for 10 minutes. Add other ingredients, tomatoes, and remaining broth.

Boil, cover, and simmer for about 3 hours.

When beans are soft and liquid is absorbed, they are done. Makes 6 portions. (1 portion = 304.1 calories, 3.2 grams fat,   22% protein,   69% carbohydrates, 9% fat)

Barbecue Baked Beans

1C	Onion, diced
3	cans Beans (14-16 oz. kidney, black, navy, pinto, great northern, lima)
2 Tbsp.	Blackstrap molasses
2 Tbsp.	Apple cider vinegar
1 Tbsp.	Dry mustard
½ tsp.	Garlic powder
½C	Tomato ketchup
	Canola oil cooking spray

Heat oven to 350o F. While heating, sauté onion in an oil-sprayed nonstick pan. Pour off half the liquid from each bean can. Mix beans and remaining ingredients in large bowl and add onion. Mix thoroughly. Put into a 2-quart casserole and bake, uncovered, for 1½ hours, stirring after 1 hour. Makes 4 to 6 portions. (1 portion = 279.1 calories, 1.6 grams fat, 18% protein, 77% carbohydrates, 5% fat)

Quick Chili

4 cloves	Garlic, chopped
½C	Onion, chopped
1-2 Tbsp.	Chili powder
2 cans	Kidney beans (14 oz. size, with liquid from 1 can only or sauce will be too thin)
1 can	Tomato sauce (8 oz.)
¼ tsp.	Cumin

Sauté garlic and onions in water in a dutch oven. Add chili powder. Add kidney beans and tomato sauce. Simmer for 30 minutes. Makes 4 to 6 portions. (1 portion = 159.2 calories, 1.0 grams fat, 23% protein, 72% carbohydrates, 5% fat)

Sweet and Sour Tofu

Sauce:

1 lb.	Tofu, cut into 1½" pieces
¾C	Water
2/3 C	Honey
2 Tbsp.	Corn starch
2 Tbsp.	Soy sauce
3 Tbsp.	Rice vinegar
	Olive oil cooking spray

Lightly spray nonstick skillet, brown the tofu until golden and textured on the outside (about 5 minutes, watching carefully).

Mix sauce ingredients together and pour over tofu, stirring constantly until sauce thickens.

Cover and simmer for 30 minutes. Makes 4 portions. (1 portion = 259.2 calories, 3.3 grams fat, 12% protein, 78% carbohydrates, 11% fat)

Tomato, green pepper, pineapple chunks, cilantro, and toasted sesame seeds make excellent garnishes.

Chickenless Long Rice

This is a variation on the traditional lu'au-style chicken long rice. It can be done with or without chicken. Both can be low-fat selections if prepared properly. Everyone should try this at least once to see that it can be tasty either way.

1/2 tsp.	Sesame oil
1 large	Round onion, diced
3 cloves	Garlic, crushed
2 quarts	Water
3 Tbsp.	Chicken-flavored vegetarian broth (instant)
1" piece	Ginger root, peeled and crushed
8 oz.	Long rice
1/2 C	Shiitake mushrooms (dried), soaked, sliced
1/2 C	Green onions

Soak shiitake mushrooms in water to cover for 10 to 15 minutes. Drain, slice, and set aside. Soak long rice in water to cover for 10 to 15 minutes. Sauté onion and garlic in sesame oil until onions are slightly browned. Add water, instant broth mix, and gin- ger; simmer together at least 10 minutes. Drain long rice and cut into 3" lengths. Add to broth and cook until noodles are done. Add shiitake mushrooms and stir. Garnish with green onions and serve.

Makes 6 portions. (1 portion = 173 calories, 0.5 gram fat, 7% protein, 90% carbohydrates, 3% fat)

Srambled Tofu

Scrambled Tofu is a delicious substitute for scrambled eggs. The best reason to replace eggs for breakfast is the 430 mg. of cholesterol found in two eggs (more than the amount of cholesterol in an 8-ounce steak). Tofu, of course, as in any plant-based product,
has no cholesterol.

1 block	Tofu, firm
1/4 C	Onions, minced
2 tsp.	Vegetarian "chicken-flavored" seasoning
1/2 tsp.	Turmeric
1/4 tsp.	Sea salt
1/4 tsp.	Onion powder
1/4 tsp.	Garlic powder
	Canola oil cooking spray

Lightly spray a large non-stick skillet with canola oil cooking spray. Sauté onions, adding a slight amount of water if they start to stick. As the onions cook, add sea- sonings and mix.

Break up tofu into scrambled-egg consistency and add to the mixture. Cook until the mixture is thoroughly heated and resembles scrambled eggs.

Serve with whole grain toast or pancakes.
Makes 5 portions. (1 portion = 95 calories, 4.2 grams fat, 38% protein, 24% carbohydrates, 38% fat)

Tofu Nuggets

1 blk.	Firm tofu, cut in ¾" cubes
1/3 C	Nutritional yeast
1 tsp.	Spike® seasoning or vegetarian chicken broth powder
½ tsp.	Black pepper
1½ Tbsp.	Soy sauce or tamari
¼ tsp.	Olive or sesame oil (or cooking spray)

Slice or break tofu into approximately ¾" cubes. Coat nonstick pan with oil or cooking spray and heat at medium-high. Add tofu cubes and brown. Turn heat to low and drizzle soy sauce on each piece of tofu. Add yeast, Spike®, and pepper and toss, coating the pieces of tofu evenly. Cook until golden brown. Makes 2 to 4 portions. (1 portion = 118.2 calories, 3.6 grams fat, 45% protein, 29% carbohydrates, 26% fat)

Broiled Falafel

2C   Garbanzo beans, cooked (¾ C dry)
½C   Parsley clusters

Put in mixing bowl with:

3 cloves   Garlic, pressed
2 Tbsp.   Egg replacer
½ tsp.   Dry mustard
1 tsp.   Cumin
½ tsp.   Chili powder
                Celery salt, to taste
                Salt and pepper, to taste
1tsp.   Worcestershire™ sauce
2-3   Pita pocket bread

Purée garbanzo beans and parsley in blender. Mix blended beans with all other ingredients.

Place on a lightly oil-sprayed baking pan.
Spread mixture on broiler pan, broil, and toss every 10 minutes.
Fill ½ pita pocket bread with falafel, lettuce, tomato, onion, and salsa. Makes 4 to 6 portions.   (1 portion = 206.4 calories, 2.7 grams fat, 19% protein, 69% carbohydrates, 11% fat)

Hawaiian Savory Stew

This dish was so well liked despite the fact that it had no meat in it that it was published in the newspapers. You'll be pleasantly surprised at its authentic local flavor.

3 Tbsp.	Water
1 large	Onion, chopped
2 cloves	Garlic, minced
1 piece	Ginger (1"), mashed
1 box	Seitan (wheat gluten), cut in 1" pieces or 1 C mushrooms
1 Tbsp.	Soy sauce
2 large	Carrots, cut in 1" chunks 2 stalks Celery, cut in 1" chunks
3	Red potatoes,
1 can	quartered Tomatoes, whole packed
3	Bay leaves
2C	Vegetable broth Water, to cover
	Salt, to taste
	Pepper, to taste
2 Tbsp.	Whole wheat flour dissolved in
4 Tbsp.	water

Tabasco® sauce (optional)
Sauté onion and garlic in 3 tablespoons of water in a large pot. Add seitan or mushrooms, ginger, soy sauce, carrots, celery, potatoes, tomatoes, vegetable broth, water to cover, salt, pepper, and bay leaves. Cook until vegetables are tender. Thicken with whole wheat flour dissolved in 4 tablespoons of water.

Serve hot. Zing it with a few drops of Tabasco® sauce.
Makes 6 to 8 portions. (1 portion (with seitan) = 256 calories, 1.2
grams fat, 32% protein, 64% carbohydrates, 4% fat)
(1 portion (with mushrooms) = 132 calories, 0.5 gram fat, 17%
protein, 80% carbohydrates, 3% fat)

Red Chili Lentil Stew

Chef Roy Yamaguchi contributed this spicy, versatile recipe. It can be served as a hot, hearty soup; as a side dish or as a condiment for broiled fish it takes on quite a different flavor. I have modified it slightly to reduce the fat content.

1C	Red or brown lentils
1 Tbsp.	Olive oil
1	Onion, finely diced
1-1/2 Tbsp.	Garlic, minced
2 Tbsp.	Carrot, finely diced
3	Bay leaves
2 Tbsp.	Celery, finely diced
1 tsp.	Red chili flakes (dried), crushed
1 lb.	Tomatoes, peeled, seeded, and diced
2C	Vegetarian chicken broth
1-1/2 C	Tomato juice (canned)
2 tsp.	Basil (fresh), julienned
1 tsp.	Thyme (fresh), minced
1 tsp.	Tarragon (fresh), minced
1 Tbsp.	Salt
1/2 tsp.	Sugar
1/2 tsp.	Pepper, freshly ground

VINAIGRETTE:

1/2 Tbsp.	Sherry Vinegar
1 tsp.	Olive oil

In a colander wash lentils under a cold tap. Then soak in a bowl of water for half an hour, drain, and set aside.

In a colander wash lentils under a cold tap. Then soak in a bowl of water for half an hour, drain, and set aside.

Heat the olive oil in a large stockpot, and sauté the onion, garlic, carrot, and celery over high heat about 1 to 2 minutes or until mix is lightly browned. Now stir in the rest of the ingredients except the lentils, sherry vine- gar, and remaining olive oil. Continue to stir for about a minute, and then add the lentils. Cook over medium heat for about 30 minutes, or until the lentils are just tender, but before they get mushy.

Whisk together the vinaigrette ingredients just before serving, and stir it into the lentil stew.

Variation:
To prepare this stew as a side dish or a condiment,
cut the ingredient quantities in half and omit the vinaigrette. Cook as above, then strain the lentils and reserve the liquid. Spread the lentils on a baking sheet, then refrigerate. Serve cold, or you may warm the lentils in a saucepan along with a little of the reserved liquid. Makes 6 portions.   (1 portion as entrée = 127 calories, 3.4 grams fat, 20% protein, 57% carbohydrates, 22% fat) (1 por- tion as side dish = 60 calories, 1.3 grams fat, 21% protein, 60% carbohydrates, 18% fat)

Vegetable Stew

This is a variation on a meatless stew that has a nice Mediterranean flavor to it.

1 tsp.	Extra virgin olive oil
1 large	Red onion, halved and sliced
2 cloves	Garlic, chopped 1 large Red bell pepper
1-2/3 C	Tomatoes with juice, crushed, canned
1 large	Carrot, cut into 1" pieces
1 small	Eggplant
3/4 C	Water
2	Potatoes, cut into 1" pieces
2	Zucchini, thickly sliced
4 oz.	Peas
4 oz.	Garbanzo beans
1C	Green beans, cut
1 tsp.	Salt
1 tsp.	Pepper

In a large saucepan brown the garlic and onion in hot oil. Add red bell pepper and cook for 2 minutes. Add tomatoes and cook for 2 more minutes. Add car- rots, eggplant, and water and cook for 2 more minutes. Add potatoes, zucchini, peas, beans, green beans, salt, and pepper and cook for 20 minutes or until potatoes are cooked. Serve hot or cold.
Makes 6 portions.   (1 portion = 175 calories, 2.1 grams fat, 19% protein, 71% carbohydrates, 10% fat)

Vegetable Laulau

This meatless variation of the typical pork laulau was used in the last week of the Hawaii Health Program which was a vegetarian week.

1 lb.	Sweet potatoes 1 lb. Taro
8 - 12	Ti leaves
1 lb.	Taro (lu'au) leaves, (if unavailable, use spinach leaves)
	Salt, to taste

Cut taro stems from taro leaves. Wash taro leaves.
Separate into four portions.
Taro and taro leaves must be cooked properly. Do NOT eat raw.
For more information see pages 55 and 189.
Wash and scrub taro and sweet potatoes thoroughly until clean.
Peel and cut into 1/2" cubes.
Place portions of sweet potatoes and taro on taro leaves; salt to taste. Wrap in ti leaves. Steam in pressure cooker for 20 to 25 minutes or until done.

Variation:
You can cook other vegetables in this manner such
as carrots, white potatoes, squash, etc.
In case you don't already know, the ti leaf is the traditional laulau wrapper, but is itself inedible.

Makes 4 portions. (1 portion = 264 calories, 0.8 gram fat, 10% protein, 88% carbohydrates, 2% fat)

Maui Tacos Black Bean Burrito

One of my assistants asserts that caffeine and newsprint make a complete protein. This is not so. However, rice and beans, the daily fare of Latin Americans, do make a healthy combination. Add some potatoes and enjoy this hearty burrito recipe contributed by Chef Mark Ellman of Avalon and Maui Tacos restaurants. If you want this made for you, go to one of the Maui Tacos locations in Napili, Lahaina, Kihei, Kahului, Hilo, and Honolulu.

12 oz.	Rice, cooked or Spanish rice
5 small	Potatoes
1/2	Onion, chopped
1 Tbsp.	Garlic (granulated)
1 tsp.	Salt
1 can	Black beans (16 oz.), or cooked
5	Tortillas (12")
8 oz.	Lettuce, shredded
7 oz.	Salsa or Maui Tacos' Pineapple Tomatillo Salsa
4 oz.	Maui Tacos' Guacamole

Wash and peel potatoes. Place in saucepan and water to cover. Add salt. Boil potatoes for 35 to 40 minutes. Drain water and cube into 1/2" cubes and set aside. Water-sauté onion and granulated garlic until translucent. Add black beans, potatoes, and rice. Gently mix together until combined. Lay out tortillas on a flat surface. Layer the filling in the following order: black bean-potato-rice mixture, lettuce, salsa, and guacamole. Fold tortilla over layers, envelope fashion. Makes 5 portions. (1 portion with guacamole = 440 calories, 4.9 grams fat, 13% protein, 77% carbohydrates, 10% fat) (1 portion without guacamole = 416 calories, 2.7 grams fat, 13% protein, 81% carbohydrates, 6% fat)

Dick Allgire's Lazy Enchiladas

Television newsman Dick Allgire, who contributed this recipe, says: "I call these 'Lazy Enchiladas' because the sauce and filling are cooked in the same pot and there is no baking time. With tomato on the inside, it has a nice creamy texture that I missed when giving up cheese. The spices are approximate because I don't measure; just taste until it's right."

1 medium	Onion, chopped
1/2 medium	Red/green pepper, chopped
2 cloves	Garlic, minced (bottled)
9-10 medium	Mushrooms, sliced thinly
1 can	Stewed tomatoes (15 oz.), with juice
1/2 C	Corn kernels (frozen), thawed
1 can	Black beans (15 oz.), rinsed
1/2 tsp.	Cinnamon
1/2 tsp.	Oregano, or to taste
2 Tbsp. or to taste	Cumin (ground), or to taste
1-2 tsp.	Chili powder,
pinch	Cayenne, or to taste
4 medium	Flour tortillas

Water-sauté onion, pepper, and garlic until onion is translucent. Add spices and let them coat the onion mixture. Add mushrooms and let cook briefly for 1 to 2 minutes. Add can of stewed tomatoes and bring to a simmer, reduce heat and simmer for 10 minutes. Add corn and simmer for 10 more minutes. Add beans, and simmer for 5 minutes. Warm tortillas so they are pliable, and with a slotted spoon scoop mixture in tortilla, roll, and place on dinner plate. With tablespoon, take liquid and pour over tortillas. Repeat until done. Simmering times are approximate, but essentially you want to let it cook so the flavors have combined, but not to reduce to a true stew. It should look like a soupy stew, so that you have liquid to put on tortillas.

Makes 4 portions. (1 portion = 316 calories, 3.5 grams fat, 18% protein, 72% carbohydrates, 10% fat)

Ann's Garbanzo Casserole

(Contributed by Ann Tang)

1/2 lb	cooked garbanzo beans
8oz can	whole tomatoes
1	Onion cut into 1/2" chunks
1	carrot, sliced
1 tsp	Basil

Soak garbanzo beans overnight in water to cover, or bring to boil, remove from heat and let rest for one hour. Saute onions and carrot sin 1/2 C water. Add soaked beans and tomatoes. Add more water to cover and add the basil. Bring to a boil, cover and simmer for at least 2 hours until garbanzos are tender.

Beans and Carrot Stew

1 C	pink beans
1 C	black turtle beans
5	fresh tomatoes, chopped
1	bell pepper, chopped
1	Anaheim pepper, chopped
	stalks celery, chopped
6	large carrots, diced
1/2	round onion, chopped
6	sprigs parsley, chopped
1-1/2 Tbsp	chili powder
1/2 tsp	paprika
1/2 tsp	oregano
1/2 tsp	summer savory
1/2	bay leaf
1 clove	garlic, minced

Saute garlic and onion in 1 cup water until transparent. Add tomatoes and beans and simmer 1 hour. Add remainder of ingredients and simmer another 30-45 minutes. Excellent with brown rice or over a baked potato. Freezes well.

Zip Burritos

4	Whole wheat tortillas or chapatis
1C	Nonfat refried beans
½C	Fresh salsa
1C	Lettuce, chopped
½C	Alfalfa sprouts
1	Tomato, chopped
1	Green onion,chopped

Heat the beans either in a microwave or put them in a saucepan, stirring them on the stove until heated. Spoon some of the nonfat refried beans onto a tortilla from end to end, then add fresh salsa (if you are in a hurry, use bottled salsa) over the beans. Next add the chopped lettuce, alfalfa sprouts, tomatoes, and green onion. Fold in the sides of the tortilla and hold it together with a toothpick. Makes 4 portions.

(1 portion = 183.2 calories, 3.0 grams fat, 15% protein, 71% carbohydrates, 14% fat)

 This makes a delicious, quick burrito that you
can eat any time. You can find canned nonfat refried beans in a health food store. Make sure it says nonfat refried beans rather than low-fat, because even low-fat refried beans can contain 3 to 5 grams of fat per serving.

Pronto Bean and Rice Burritos

1C	Basmati brown rice, steamed until tender and set aside
10	Whole-wheat chapatis or tortillas
1 can	Chili beans (16 oz.),cooked
1	Bell pepper, diced
1	Tomato, chopped
¼C	Onion, chopped
1 clove	Garlic, minced
1 tsp.	Ground cumin, or to taste
1 Tbsp.	Chili powder, or to taste
2 Tbsp.	Prepared salsa
¼C Green	Onions,chopped
¼C	Cilantro, chopped

Lightly warm chapatis or tortillas in oven, watching carefully so they remain soft. Reheat rice.

In the meantime, combine beans, bean liquid, bell pepper, tomato, onion, garlic, cumin, chili powder, and salsa in a saucepan. Simmer about 5 minutes.

Place a heaping tablespoon of rice and 1 to 2 tablespoons of the bean mixture in the warm chapatis or tortilla. Garnish with additional salsa, green onions, and cilantro and roll into a burrito.

Makes 10 portions. (1 portion = 238.5 calories, 3.6 grams fat, 14% protein, 72% carbohydrates, 14% fat)

Chapati Burritos

6   Chapatis (or more)
2C   Lettuce, shredded
1C   Beans,   cooked, drained (kidneys, black, pintos)
1   Cucumber, julienned
1C   Broccoli florets, blanched
½C   Tomatoes, diced
½C   Red or green bell peppers, cut in thin strips
½C   Round and green onions, sliced very thin
¼C   Cilantro, chopped Salsa, to taste

Warm chapatis (if you use the microwave, make sure they don't get brittle). Place warm chapati on plate.

Build burrito with above condiments, starting with lettuce and ending with the salsa.

 Roll and enjoy! Makes 6 portions. (1 portion = 150.8 calories, 1.3 grams fat, 18% protein, 75% carbohydrates, 7% fat)

Fresh Salsa Caliente

1	Jalapeño or other small green chili peppers, seeded and coarsely chopped Cayenne pepper(optional, to taste)
4-6 cloves	Garlic, minced
5 small	Ripe Roma tomatoes, cored and coarsely chopped
2 Tbsp.	Fresh lime juice
½ med.	Onion, minced
½ tsp.	Cumin, ground
1 tsp.	Chili powder
½	Bell pepper, minced
¼C	Cilantro, chopped
2 Tbsp.	Parsley, minced
½ tsp.	Black pepper
1 tsp.	Garlic salt

Mix ingredients, marinate in refrigerator for 12 hours. Will keep, refrigerated, for 4 to 5 days. Makes 8 portions (about 2 cups). (1 portion = 25.0 calories, 0.3 grams fat, 15% protein,   76% carbohydrates, 9% fat)

Mock Tuna

(made w/garbanzo beans)

1   15-oz. can organic garbanzo beans (drained)

Mash garbanzos (fork or potato masher will do if only making a small amount). You may still want to use a food processor to speed up your mashing. Mix following ingredients with beans while mashing:

1/4 tsp	salt
2 tsp	lemon juice
1/4 tsp	pepper
1 tsp	soy sauce
1/2 tsp	Kelp powder
1/2 tsp	Spike Seasoning

(Kelp powder can be purchased at Down to Earth spice jar counter)

After mashing, then add following ingredients and mix well. (Do not food-process beans with these ingredients---just mix it in.)

1/4 Cup	Minced celery
1 Tblspn	Minced round onions or green onions (sliced ft
2 Tblspn	Nutritional yeast
1/2Cup	Fat Free Nayonaise (or other Fat Free vegan mayo)

Use in sandwiches, salads, or as a dip.

Bean Dips

Bean dips are one of my personal favorites because they are so versatile. I love to use them to replace high-fat dips. They are also tasty, low in fat, and can be used for snack foods as well as sandwiches. A variety of beans can be used in dips and spreads, depending on your personal taste. My favorite happens to be garbanzo bean dip. This is also known as a Mediterranean dish called hummus. If you want a bean dip that is even more convenient, use non- fat refried beans straight from the can to use as a dip or to spread on your sandwiches (in addition to its more common use in burritos and tostadas).

EMWL Bean Dip

2	Onions, raw, chopped
3 cloves	Garlic, crushed
1 can	Tomatoes
2 cans	Black beans (15 oz.), drained
1 Tbsp.	Chili powder
1 Tbsp.	Chili con carne seasoning
2 tsp.	Cumin
2 tsp.	Coriander
¼ tsp.	Cayenne

Sauté onions and garlic in nonstick pan with a touch of water, until soft. Add beans, heat through, move to blender and blend to dip consistency. Add spices and continue to blend until thoroughly mixed.

Use with low-fat crackers, chips, or spread onto a burrito or taco to make a bean base for your Mexican treats. You can be creative with this dip. Some people prefer to use fresh cooked beans; others like the speed of using canned. You can add chopped tomato, pepper, more onion, whatever suits your taste. Makes 6 portions. (1 portion = 225.7 calories, 1.4 grams fat, 24% protein, 71% carbohydrates, 5% fat)

Black Bean Dip

1 can	Black beans (15 oz.) plus ½ C liquid from can
¼C	Tomato-based salsa
¼C	Onion, diced
2 cloves	Garlic, roughly chopped

Mix all ingredients together and simmer until most of the liquid has evaporated. Puree and set aside. Makes 6 portions.

(1 portion = 99.2 calories, 0.4 grams   fat,   25%   protein, 71% carbohydrates, 3% fat)

Simple Hummus

1C	Garbanzo beans, cooked
2-3 Tbsp.	Lemon juice
1 Tbsp.	Onion, minced
1 clove	Garlic, crushed
1 tsp.	Cumin
	Low-sodium soy sauce or salt, to taste
	Pepper to taste
	Water
1 tsp	Ground up sesame seeds

Cook the dry garbanzo beans per package directions. (Also, see bean cooking chart on page 308.) You may use precooked canned beans instead, if you wish. Mash beans and mix ingredients together with enough water to keep a thick moist dip consistency. Makes 8 portions.

(1 portion = 93.5 calories, 1.3 grams fat, 22% protein, 67% carbohydrates, 12% fat)

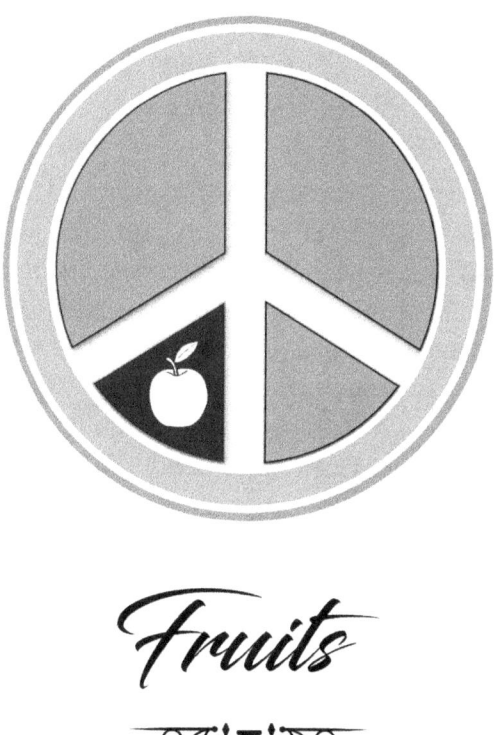

Fruits

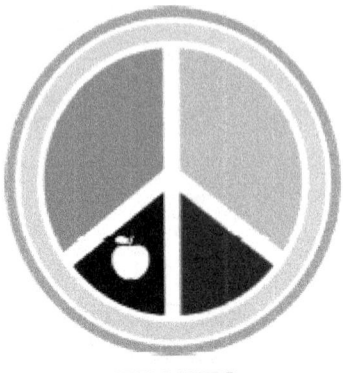

FRUITS

Most fruits are high on the SMI scale and as a result will not contribute to weight gain. They also contain a wealth of vitamins and phytonutrients such as beta- carotene and vitamin C. But fruit has relatively high sugar content. Fructose, the natural sugar in fruit, can be absorbed very quickly. It's not as bad as white sugar, but it's still not good for you in large amounts. As with processed sugars, it tends to cause a rise in triglycerides (storage fats) in our blood. High triglycerides are a co-risk factor with cholesterol for heart disease.

Have a piece of raw fruit, such as an orange, apple, blueberries or other treat, either as a snack or for breakfast. It's portable, so very convenient as a snack or a breakfast on the go. Use fruits as a dessert to satisfy your sweet tooth, but don't eat too much fruit. Two to four servings is fine for most people. Fruit – easy access and easier preparation. Yet, research shows that, even though people who eat fruit regularly have reduced rates of all cancers, heart disease, and other illnesses, half of all Americans don't eat fruit at all. Moderation is the key here.

Eating the whole fruit is better than drinking fruit juice or consuming fruit smoothies. Liquefying fruit or any food tends to raise the glycemic index of the food. In other words, processing the food tends to increase its rate of absorption and raises blood sugar levels and insulin requirement. Some people find that fruits are easier to digest if they are cooked. Others do better with raw fruit. Some people go on "fruit fasts" as an effective way to lose weight. I don't recommend this approach. It would cause weight loss, because fruits are high on the SMI. But I believe a more balanced diet is important for good health. If possible, try to eat fruit in season, and from your own locality.

Apple-Strawberry Jel

It surprises many people to learn that most gelatin is made from animals' collagen, which is a protein derived from boiling down the joints and tendons of animals such as cows. While this is a non-fat, non-cholesterol product, it is made of animal protein. Another problem with commercial gelatins is that they are usually artificially colored and contain a great deal of sugar. A far better alternative is agar (also called agar-agar). This is a form of seaweed which provides a gelling effect. I use natural fruit and fruit juices for the sweetening. Agar gelatin is just as easy to prepare as commercial gelatins, and it has a better flavor because natural foods are used.

8 Tbsp.	Agar flakes
6C	Apple juice
1 pint	Strawberries
½C	Apples, cut into very small chunks

Mix agar, juice, and water in a saucepan, bring to a boil then simmer 4 to 5 minutes until dissolved.

Wash, clean, and slice strawberries. Clean and cut apples. Use a fancy gelatin mold in a fruit shape if you have one. Otherwise, line the bottom of a 9" shallow rectangular baking

169

pan with two-thirds of the strawberries, setting the remainder aside. Add a small layer of apples.

Gently pour the hot agar mixture over the fruits in the first pan to a depth of about 1". Pour any remaining agar mixture over fruits in the second pan. Chill until firmly set. To serve, slice into appropriate serving sizes. Blend the mixture that has set in the second dish until smooth. Serve as a sauce over the molded gelatin slices or squares. Makes 4 portions. (1 portion = 218.4 calories, 0.3 grams fat, 1% protein, 97% carbohydrates, 1% fat)

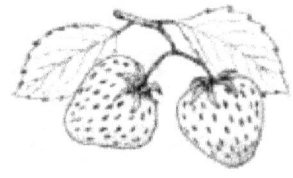

Baked Apple With Raisin Sauce

5	Apples, any variety (Rome, Pippin, Granny Smith, or Jonathan are good baking apples)
1 Tbsp.	Arrowroot or cornstarch
1C	Apple juice
1 tsp.	Cinnamon
¼C	Raisins
½ tsp.	Vanilla

Preheat oven to 375 °F. Wash apples, cut off the top, and core into the apple about halfway down to get the seeds out but do not poke through the bottom.

Place into a baking pan with a small amount of water and bake for 15 to 20 minutes. Place apple juice, raisins, cinnamon, vanilla and a pinch of salt into a saucepan and bring to a boil. Then simmer at low heat for 5 minutes. Dissolve the arrowroot in cool water and add to mixture and stir. Spoon sauce into the apples and enjoy. Makes 5 portions. (1 portion = 126.7 calories, 0.449 grams fat, 1% protein, 96% carbohydrates, 3% fat)

Peach Crisp

Filling:

4C	Canned sliced peaches in juice
3 Tbsp.	Whole wheat flour
1/8 C	Fruit-juice-sweetened apricot preserves
4 Tbsp.	Honey
2 tsp.	Lemon juice
1/8 tsp.	Nutmeg

Topping:

1 Tbsp.	Maple syrup
½ tsp.	Vanilla
¼C	Whole oats
1 Tbsp.	Cornmeal
¼ tsp.	Cinnamon

Fold peaches into flour and pour mixture into a 9" pie pan. Mix preserves with honey, lemon juice, and nutmeg. Spoon mixture over peaches and bake at 375o F. for 30 minutes. Take out of oven. Mix toppings. Crumble over peach filling. Bake for 15 moreminutes. Makes 8 portions. (1 portion = 128.5 calories, 0.5grams fat, 6% protein, 91% carbohydrates, 3% fat)

Quick Apple Pie

½C	Grape Nuts® cereal
4C	Delicious apples (large)
2 tsp.	Cinnamon
2 tsp.	Corn starch
2 tsp.	Lemon juice
1/3 C	Frozen apple juice concentrate, thawed
½ tsp.	Ground coriander
¼C	Raisins

Preheat the oven to 400o F.
Core the apples, slice thin,
and sprinkle with lemon juice.
Blend Grape Nuts®, pulsing
until it's almost pulverized. Spread
over the bottom of a covered casserole
dish. Dissolve corn starch in 1/3 cup
of apple juice and cook until thick.
Mix apples, juice, and spices in a bowl.
Spread the apple mixture over the cereal in the
casserole dish.   Sprinkle   with   additional   cinnamon,   if
desired.
Cover and bake for 45 minutes, or until apples are tender.
Remove cover and return to oven to allow pie to brown for 10 to
15 minutes longer. Makes 6 portions.

(1 portion = 127.5 calories, 0.4 grams fat, 5% protein, 93%
carbohydrates, 3% fat)

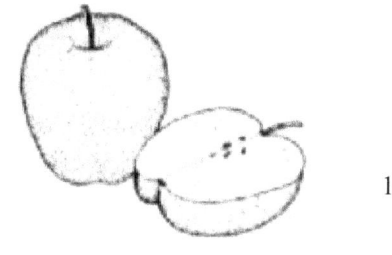

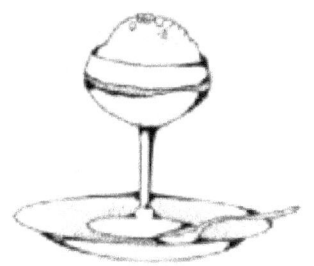

Iced Fruit Cream

SOME FACTS: Desserts can be festive and healthy if you use just a little bit of imagination. One of the best desserts I ever tasted was frozen bananas run through a Champion® juicer or a Yonanna® .. This produces a consistency very much like soft-serve ice cream. If you add just a hint of vanilla you'll actually get a very tasty ice creamy product, though it's really not necessary. In fact, you can use frozen bananas as a base and then add frozen strawberries, or any other flavor by adding a frozen version of the fruit to the banana mixture.

4C   Bananas, frozen
1/2 C   Other fruit of your choice ie strawberry, blueberry, etc, frozen.

Put 4" segments of frozen bananas pieces in the blender with ¼ cup water or juice. Add more liquid if needed. Blend smooth. Serve immediately. Makes 8 portions. (1 portion = 111.5 calories, 0.581   grams fat,   4%   protein,   92% carbohydrates, 4% fat)

Top with fresh banana slices, nuts, or cherries. Add other fruits as desired, or no-sugar- added extracts such as strawberries, blueberries, pears, vanilla, maple, and almond.

A Few More Sweet Delights

Strawberry-Banana Pudding

1½ C	Low-fat firm tofu (Mori Nu firm tofu is suggested)
1½ C	Fresh strawberries, sliced
1	Banana
1 tsp.	Vanilla
1 Tbsp.	Lemon juice
¼ tsp.	Salt
2 Tbsp.	Honey

Blend all ingredients together in blender or food processor until creamy and smooth. Pour into individual serving dishes, or pour into individual-sized Grape Nuts® pie shells (make by putting muffin cups in muffin pan then pouring in Grape Nuts®). Chill overnight. Makes 4 to 6 portions. (1 portion = 109.4 calories, 1.886 grams fat, 23% protein, 62% carbohydrates, 15% fat)

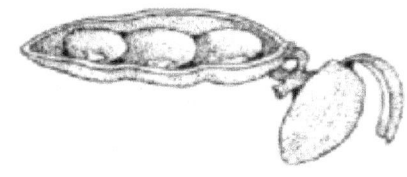

Honey Almond Fruit Cocktail

1C	Watermelon
1C	Honeydew melon
1C	Apple
½C	Cantaloupe or pineapple chunks
1	Peach or pear
6 Tbsp.	Agar
2C	Water
1C	Unsweetened soy milk
3 Tbsp.	Honey Almond extract, to taste

Dissolve agar in water, heat.

When completely dissolved, add soy milk, honey, and almond extract, to taste.

Cool and let set. Cut into small chunks.

Cut watermelon, honeydew melon, apple, cantaloupe, and peach or pear into ½" chunks.

Mix agar chunks together with chunks of various fruits for an unusual and colorful fruit cocktail. Makes 8 portions.

(1 portion = 84.72 calories, 0.588 grams fat, 7% protein, 87% carbohydrates, 6% fat)

GLYCEMIC INDEX (GI) AND

DR. SHINTANI'S

FOOD MASS INDEX (SMI) TABLES

Glycemic Index. (GI) - Lower is better.

The glycemic index is an index of numbers that represent how high blood sugar will rise in response to the consumption of a specific food. The higher the number, the higher the blood sugar will rise.   It is based on studies of the blood sugar response in normal non-diabetic people when they eat 50 grams of carbohydrate from a specific food. The number is derived by comparing this blood sugar rise to a standard food. The GI(glu) column is a table of numbers comparing blood sugar rise of a food compared to how high blood sugar rises compared to glucose. The GI(bread) column is the blood sugar rise caused by a food compared to how high blood sugar rises compared to white bread. Thus, a food with a lower GI number is preferred.

The Shintani Mass Index (SMI) - Higher is better

The SMI table is the "Shintani Mass Index" which is a table based on the number of pounds required of a specific food to provide one day's worth of calories. It is based on 2500 calories which is an estimated amount of calories for an average man or average active woman. So, for example, the SMI number of apple is 9.6 which means it takes 9.6 pounds of apples to provide 2500 calories or one day's worth of calories. The SMI of boiled potato is 6.4. the SMI value of potato chips is 1.0. This means that it takes 6.4 pounds of boiled potato for a day's worth of calories but only 1 pound of potato chips. You can see that apples or boiled potato will fill your stomach faster than potato chips and you will wind up eating fewer calories if the SMI number is high. An SMI number higher than 4 is considered good because studies show that most people will not eat more than 4.1 pounds of food per day. Thus, a food with a higher SMI number is preferred.

GLYCEMIC INDEX (GI) AND DR.SHINTANI'S FOOD MASS INDEX (SMI)			
Food Item	**GI (glu)**	**GI (bread)**	**Mass Index**
All-Bran®, Kellogg's	42	60	1.4
Angel food cake	67	96	2.1
Apple, dried	29	41	4.6
Apple, fresh	36	51	9.6
Apricot jam	55	79	2.0
Apricots, canned, light syrup	64	91	8.7
Apricots, dried	31	44	4.6
Apricots, fresh	57	81	10.4
Asparagus	*	*	21
Avocado	*	*	3.3
Bacon	*	*	0.8
Bagel, white, frozen	72	103	2.0
Baked beans	48	69	5.1
Banana	53	76	6.0
Banana bread	47	67	1.7
Barley, cracked	50	71	4.5
Barley, pearled	25	36	4.5
Beans, Black	30	43	4.2
Beans, green	*	*	21.9
Beans, Lentils	*	*	5.2
Beans, mung spr	*	*	15.6
Beef, Corned	*	*	1.5
Beef, Ground	*	*	1.9
Beef, steak	*	*	1.2
Beets	64	91	17.8
Black-eyed peas	42	60	5.1
Blueberry Muffin	59	84	2.0
Bran Buds®, Kellogg's	58	83	1.4
Bran Chex®, Nabisco	58	83	1.2
Bran Flakes®, Post	74	106	1.7
Bread stuffing	74	106	2.1
Breadfruit	68	97	4.6

*GI cannot be calculated on some foods because of insufficient carbohydrate in them

GLYCEMIC INDEX (GI) AND DR.SHINTANI'S FOOD MASS INDEX (SMI)			
Food Item	**GI (glu)**	**GI (bread)**	**Mass Index**
BREADS			
Bagel, white, frozen	72	103	2.0
Bread stuffing	74	106	2.1
Bulgur (cracked wheat) bread	58	83	2.2
Corn tortilla	38	54	2.5
Croissant	67	96	1.4
French baguette	95	136	2.0
Hamburger bun	61	87	1.9
Kaiser roll	73	104	1.9
Melba Toast, Old London®	70	100	1.4
Mixed grain bread	45	64	1.9
Oat bran bread	47	67	1.8
Pita bread, white	57	81	2.3
Pumpernickel bread, whole grain	51	73	2.2
Rye bread	65	93	2.4
Rye bread, American light	68	97	1.9
Rye bread, dark	76	109	2.2
Sourdough bread	52	74	2.1
Stone ground whole wheat bread	43	61	2.1
Wheat chapatti	27	39	3.2
White bread	70	100	2.1
Whole wheat bread	69	99	2.2
BREAKFAST CEREALS			
All-Bran®, Kellogg's	42	60	1.4
Bran Buds®, Kellogg's	58	83	1.4
Bran Chex®, Nabisco	58	83	1.2
Bran Flakes®, Post	74	106	1.7
Cheerios®, General Mills	74	106	1.3
Corn Bran®, Quaker	75	107	1.3
Corn Chex®, Nabisco	83	119	1.6
Corn Flakes®, Kellogg's	84	120	1.4

*GI cannot be calculated on some foods because of insufficient carbohydrate in them.

GLYCEMIC INDEX (GI) AND DR.SHINTANI'S FOOD MASS INDEX (SMI)			
	GI	GI	Mass
Food Item	(glu)	(bread)	Index
Cream of Wheat®, Instant, Nabisco	74	106	10.3
Cream of Wheat®, Nabisco	66	94	10.7
Golden Grahams®, General Mills	71	101	1.4
grape-nuts®, Post	67	96	1.1
grape-nuts Flakes®, Post	80	114	1.5
Life®, Quaker	66	94	1.4
Muesli, non-toasted	56	80	1.5
Muesli, toasted	43	61	1.5
Nutri-Grain®, Kellogg's	66	94	1.5
Oat Bran Cereal®, Quaker	50	71	1.5
Oat bran, raw	55	79	1.7
Oatmeal (porridge), old-fashioned	59	84	8.9
Oatmeal, one minute instant	66	94	8.9
Puffed Wheat®, Quaker	74	106	1.5
Rice Chex®, General Mills	89	127	1.8
Rice Krispies®, Kellogg's	82	117	1.4
Shredded Wheat®, Nabisco	69	99	1.5
Special K®, Kellogg's	54	77	1.4
Team Flakes®, Nabisco	82	117	1.4
Total®, General Mills	76	109	1.6
Wheat cereal	41	59	9.7
Wheat cereal, quick cooking	54	77	9.1
Broad beans	79	113	7.7
Broccoli	*	*	17.1
Buckwheat	54	77	6.0
Bulgur wheat	48	69	6.6
Bulgur (cracked wheat) bread	58	83	2.2
Butter	*	*	0.8
Butter beans	31	44	6.7
Cabbage	*	*	22.8
Cabbage, Chinese	*	*	39

*GI cannot be calculated on some foods because of insufficient carbohydrate in them.

GLYCEMIC INDEX (GI) AND DR.SHINTANI'S FOOD MASS INDEX (SMI)			
	GI	GI	Mass
Food Item	(glu)	(bread)	Index
CAKE			
Angel food cake	67	96	2.1
Banana bread	47	67	1.7
Pound cake	54	77	0.9
Sponge cake	46	66	1.9
CANDY			
Chocolate candy	49	70	1.1
Jelly beans	80	114	2.3
Life Savers®	70	100	1.4
Mars Chocolate Almond Bar®, M&M Mars	68	97	1.2
M&M Chocolate Covered Peanuts®	33	47	1.1
Snickers®, M&M Mars	41	59	1.2
Twix®, Caramel, M&M Mars	44	63	1.1
Cantaloupe	65	93	15.5
Carrots	71	101	12.7
Cashew nuts	*	*	1
Cauliflower	*	*	20.2
Cheerios®, General Mills	74	106	1.3
Cherries	22	31	7.6
Cheese, Cheddar	*	*	1.4
Chicken, dark	*	*	3.1
Chicken, Fried	*	*	2.2
Chicken, white	*	*	3.3
Chocolate candy	49	70	1.1
Collards	*	*	12.1
COOKIES			
Oatmeal cookie	55	79	1.2
Shortbread cookie	64	91	1.1
Social Tea Biscuits®, Nabisco	55	79	1.4
Vanilla wafers	77	110	1.2
Corn	55	79	5.5
Corn Bran®, Quaker	75	107	1.3

*GI cannot be calculated on some foods because of insufficient carbohydrate in them.

GLYCEMIC INDEX (GI) AND DR.SHINTANI'S FOOD MASS INDEX (SMI)			
	GI	GI	Mass
Food Item	(glu)	(bread)	Index
Corn Chex®, Nabisco	83	119	1.6
Corn chips	73	104	1.0
Corn Flakes®, Kellogg's	84	120	1.4
Corn tortilla	38	54	2.5
Cornmeal	68	97	1.5
Couscous	65	93	4.9
Crab	*	*	5.9
Crab Salad	*	*	3.8
CRACKERS			
Graham crackers	74	106	1.4
Rice cakes	82	117	4.4
Rye crispbread, high fiber	65	93	1.4
Soda crackers	72	103	1.3
Stoned wheat thins	67	96	1.5
Wheat Crackers®, Breton	67	96	1.1
Cream cheese	*	*	1.5
Cream of Wheat®, Instant, Nabisco	74	106	10.3
Cream of Wheat®, Nabisco	66	94	10.7
Croissant	67	96	1.4
Cucumbers	*	*	32.8
Dates	103	147	4.0
Doughnut, cake-type	76	109	1.3
Eggplant	*	*	28.8
Eggs	*	*	3.4
Fava beans	79	113	6.9
Fettucini, egg-enriched	32	46	3.9
Fish sticks	38	54	2.0
French baguette	95	136	2.0
French fries	23	33	1.4
Fructose	23	33	1.4

*GI cannot be calculated on some foods because of insufficient carbohydrate in them.

Food Item	GI (glu)	GI (bread)	Mass Index
GLYCEMIC INDEX (GI) AND DR.SHINTANI'S FOOD MASS INDEX (SMI)			
FRUIT AND FRUIT PRODUCTS			
Apple			
Apple, dried	29	41	4.6
Apple, fresh	36	51	9.6
Apricots			
Apricot jam	55	79	2.0
Apricots, canned, light syrup	64	91	8.7
Apricots, dried	31	44	4.6
Apricots, fresh	57	81	10.4
Banana	53	76	6.0
Breadfruit	68	97	4.6
Cantaloupe	65	93	15.5
Cherries	22	31	7.6
Dates	103	147	4.0
Fruit cocktail, canned, light syrup	55	79	17.2
Grapefruit	25	36	18.3
Grapes	43	61	7.7
Kiwi	52	74	9.1
Mango	55	79	8.3
Orange	43	61	11.6
Papaya	58	83	14.3
Peach			
Peach, fresh	28	40	12.8
Peaches, canned, heavy syrup	58	83	7.4
Peaches, canned, light syrup	52	74	10.2
Peaches, canned, natural juice	30	43	12.5
Pear			
Pear, fresh	36	51	9.3
Pears, canned in pear juice, Bartlett	44	63	11.1

*GI cannot be calculated on some foods because of insufficient carbohydrate in them.

GLYCEMIC INDEX (GI) AND DR.SHINTANI'S FOOD MASS INDEX (SMI)			
Food Item	GI (glu)	GI (bread)	Mass Index
Peaches, canned, light syrup	52	74	10.2
Peaches, canned, natural juice	30	43	12.5
Pear			
Pear, fresh	36	51	9.3
Pears, canned in pear juice, Bartlett	44	63	11.1
Pineapple, fresh	66	94	11.1
Plum	24	34	10.1
Raisins	64	91	3.6
Strawberry jam	51	73	2.0
Watermelon	72	103	17.6
Fruit cocktail, canned, light syrup	55	79	17.2
Garbanzo beans, boiled (chickpeas)	33	47	5.2
Garbanzo beans, canned (chickpeas)	42	60	5.6
Glucose	97	139	1.4
Golden Grahams®, General Mills	71	101	1.4
Graham crackers	74	106	1.4
GRAINS			
Barley			
Barley, cracked	50	71	4.5
Barley, pearled	25	36	4.5
Buckwheat	54	77	6.0
Corn			
Corn	55	79	5.5
Corn chips	73	104	1.0
Corn tortilla	38	54	2.5
Cornmeal	68	97	1.5
Popcorn	55	79	1.3
Taco shells, corn	68	97	1.3
Millet	71	101	4.6

*GI cannot be calculated on some foods because of insufficient carbohydrate in them.

GLYCEMIC INDEX (GI) AND DR.SHINTANI'S FOOD MASS INDEX (SMI)			
	GI	GI	Mass
Food Item	(glu)	(bread)	Index
Oats			
Oat bran, raw	55	79	1.7
Oatmeal (porridge), old-fashioned	59	84	8.9
Oatmeal, one minute instant	66	94	8.9
Rice			
Rice, brown	55	79	4.9
Rice, instant	91	130	5.6
Rice, specialty (mixed with wild)	55	79	5.4
Rice, white (high amylose)	56	80	5.0
Rice, white, Calrose (low amylose)	83	119	4.6
Rice, white, converted	38	54	4.6
Wheat			
Bulgur wheat	48	69	6.6
Wheat cereal	41	59	9.7
Wheat cereal, quick cooking	54	77	9.1
Wheat chapatti	27	39	3.2
Grapefruit	25	36	18.3
grape-nuts®, Post	67	96	1.1
grape-nuts Flakes®, Post	80	114	1.5
Grapes	43	61	7.7
Hamb, 1/4 lb w ches	*	*	2.1
Hamburger, 1/4 lb	*	*	2.2
Hamburger bun	61	87	1.9
Ham Sandwich	*	*	1.6
Hard Candy	*	*	1.4
Honey	73	104	1.8
Instant noodles, Mr. Noodle®	47	67	4.1
Jelly beans	80	114	2.3
Kaiser roll	73	104	1.9
Kale	*	*	10.3
Kidney beans, boiled	27	39	4.3

*GI cannot be calculated on some foods because of insufficient carbohydrate in them.

GLYCEMIC INDEX (GI) AND DR.SHINTANI'S FOOD MASS INDEX (SMI)			
Food Item	GI (glu)	GI (bread)	Mass Index
Kidney beans, canned	52	74	6.1
Kiwi	52	74	9.1
Lactose	46	66	1.4
Lentils, green and brown, boiled	29	41	4.7
Life Savers®	70	100	1.4
Life®, Quaker	66	94	1.4
LEGUMES			
Baked beans	48	69	5.1
Black beans	30	43	4.2
Black-eyed peas	42	60	5.1
Broad beans	79	113	7.7
Butter beans	31	44	6.7
Fava beans	79	113	6.9
Garbanzo beans (chickpeas)			
Garbanzo beans, boiled (chickpeas)	33	47	5.2
Garbanzo beans, canned (chickpeas)	42	60	5.6
Kidney beans			
Kidney beans, boiled	27	39	4.3
Kidney beans, canned	52	74	6.1
Lentils, green and brown, boiled	29	41	4.7
Lima beans, baby, frozen	32	46	5.3
Navy (harcort) beans, boiled	38	54	3.9
Pinto beans			
Pinto beans, boiled	39	56	4.0
Pinto beans, canned	45	64	6.2
Soybeans	18	26	3.9
Split peas, yellow and green, boiled	32	46	4.7
Lemon	*	*	30.4
Lettuce	*	*	39
Lima beans, baby, frozen	32	46	5.3
Luncheon Meat	*	*	2.1

*GI cannot be calculated on some foods because of insufficient carbohydrate in them.

GLYCEMIC INDEX (GI) AND DR.SHINTANI'S FOOD MASS INDEX (SMI)

Food Item	GI (glu)	GI (bread)	Mass Index
Linguini	49	70	3.9
M&M Chocolate Covered Peanuts®	33	47	1.1
Macaroni and cheese, boxed	64	91	3.6
Macaroni, boiled 5 minutes	45	64	3.9
Maltose	105	150	1.4
Mango	55	79	8.3
Margarine	*	*	0.8
Mars Chocolate Almond Bar®, M&M Mars	68	97	1.2
Mayonnaise	*	*	0.8
Melba Toast, Old London®	70	100	1.4
Melon	*	*	18.2
Millet	71	101	4.6
Mixed grain bread	45	64	1.9
Muesli, non-toasted	56	80	1.5
Muesli, toasted	43	61	1.5
Muffin, plain	62	89	1.8
MUFFINS			
Blueberry Muffin	59	84	2.0
Muffin, plain	62	89	1.8
Oat bran muffin	60	86	2.2
Mushrooms	*	*	19.5
Mustard Greens	*	*	17.6
Navy (harcort) beans, boiled	38	54	3.9
Nutri-Grain®, Kellogg's	66	94	1.5
Oat bran bread	47	67	1.8
Oat Bran Cereal®, Quaker	50	71	1.5
Oat bran muffin	60	86	2.2
Oat bran, raw	55	79	1.7
Oatmeal cookie	55	79	1.2
Oatmeal (porridge), old-fashioned	59	84	8.9
Oatmeal, one minute instant	66	94	8.9

*GI cannot be calculated on some foods because of insufficient carbohydrate in them.

GLYCEMIC INDEX (GI) AND DR.SHINTANI'S FOOD MASS INDEX (SMI)			
Food Item	GI (glu)	GI (bread)	Mass Index
Oil/Lard	*	*	0.6
Olives	*	*	4.7
Onions	*	*	14.8
Orange	43	61	11.6
Papaya	58	83	14.3
Parsnips	97	139	6.8
PASTA			
Couscous	65	93	4.9
Fettucini, egg-enriched	32	46	3.9
Instant noodles, Mr. Noodle®	47	67	4.1
Linguini	49	70	3.9
Macaroni and cheese, boxed	64	91	3.6
Macaroni, boiled 5 minutes	45	64	3.9
Ravioli, Duram, meat-filled	39	56	4.4
Spaghetti			
Spaghetti, Duram	55	79	3.7
Spaghetti, white	41	59	3.7
Spaghetti, whole-wheat	37	53	4.4
Tortellini cheese pasta	50	71	3.3
Vermicelli	35	50	3.0
Pastry(danish)	*	*	1.5
Peach, fresh	28	40	12.8
Peaches, canned, heavy syrup	58	83	7.4
Peaches, canned, light syrup	52	74	10.2
Peaches, canned, natural juice	30	43	12.5
Peanuts	14	20	0.9
Pear, fresh	36	51	9.3
Pears, canned in pear juice, Bartlett	44	63	11.1
Peas	48	69	7.0
Pineapple, fresh	66	94	11.1
Pinto beans, boiled	39	56	4.0

*GI cannot be calculated on some foods because of insufficient carbohydrate in them.

GLYCEMIC INDEX (GI) AND DR.SHINTANI'S FOOD MASS INDEX (SMI)			
Food Item	**GI (glu)**	**GI (bread)**	**Mass Index**
Pinto beans, canned	45	64	6.2
Pita bread, white	57	81	2.3
Pizza, cheese	60	86	3.1
Plum	24	34	10.1
Poi	*	*	9.1
Popcorn	55	79	1.3
Potato, baked	85	121	5.9
Potato, boiled, mashed	73	104	6.2
Potato, canned	61	87	9.2
Potato chips	54	77	1.0
Potato, instant	83	119	7.0
Potato, new	62	89	9.1
Potato, sweet	54	77	5.3
Potato, white, baked	60	86	5.9
Potato, white, boiled	56	80	6.4
Potato, white, mashed	70	100	5.2
Potato, white, steamed	65	93	6.4
Pound cake	54	77	0.9
Puffed Wheat®, Quaker	74	106	1.5
Pumpernickel bread, whole grain	51	73	2.2
Pumpkin	75	107	16.3
Radish	*	*	32.1
Raisins	64	91	3.6
Ravioli, Duram, meat-filled	39	56	4.4
Rice, brown	55	79	4.9
Rice cakes	82	117	4.4
Rice Chex®, General Mills	89	127	1.8
Rice, instant	91	130	5.6
Rice Krispies®, Kellogg's	82	117	1.4
Rice, specialty (mixed with wild)	55	79	5.4
Rice, white (high amylose)	56	80	5.0

*GI cannot be calculated on some foods because of insufficient carbohydrate in them.

GLYCEMIC INDEX (GI) AND DR.SHINTANI'S FOOD MASS INDEX (SMI)			
Food Item	**GI (glu)**	**GI (bread)**	**Mass Index**
Rice, white, Calrose (low amylose)	83	119	4.6
Rutabaga	72	103	16.1
Rye bread	65	93	2.4
Rye bread, American light	68	97	1.9
Rye bread, dark	76	109	2.2
Rye crispbread, high fiber	65	93	1.4
Sausages	28	40	1.7
Seaweed(konbu)	*	*	12.7
Seaweed(wakame)	*	*	12.1
Shortbread cookie	64	91	1.1
Shredded Wheat®, Nabisco	69	99	1.5
Shrimp	*	*	4.8
Shrimp, Fried	*	*	2.3
SNACK FOODS			
Corn chips	73	104	1.0
Peanuts	14	20	0.9
Popcorn	55	79	1.3
Potato chips	54	77	1.0
Snickers®, M&M Mars	41	59	1.2
Social Tea Biscuits®, Nabisco	55	79	1.4
Soda crackers	72	103	1.3
Sourdough bread	52	74	2.1
Soybeans	18	26	3.9
Soybean, Sprouts	*	*	11.9
Spaghetti, Duram	55	79	3.7
Spaghetti, white	41	59	3.7
Spaghetti, whole-wheat	37	53	4.4
Special K®, Kellogg's	54	77	1.4
Spinach	*	*	21
Split peas, yellow and green, boiled	32	46	4.7
Sponge cake	46	66	1.9

*GI cannot be calculated on some foods because of insufficient carbohydrate in them.

Food Item	GI (glu)	GI (bread)	Mass Index
GLYCEMIC INDEX (GI) AND DR.SHINTANI'S FOOD MASS INDEX (SMI)			
Squash	*	*	28.8
Stone ground whole wheat bread	43	61	2.1
Stoned wheat thins	67	96	1.5
Strawberry jam	51	73	2.0
Sucrose (table sugar)	65	93	1.4
SUGARS			
Fructose	23	33	1.4
Glucose	97	139	1.4
Honey	73	104	1.8
Lactose	46	66	1.4
Maltose	105	150	1.4
Sucrose (table sugar)	65	93	1.4
Sweet Potato	*	*	5.4
Taco shells, corn	68	97	1.3
Taro	54	77	5.1
Team Flakes®, Nabisco	82	117	1.4
Tofu	*	*	7.6
Tomato	*	*	27.3
Tomato Paste	*	*	6.5
Tortellini cheese pasta	50	71	3.3
Tortilla, corn	59	84	3.0
Tortilla, flour	38	54	2.5
Total®, General Mills	76	109	1.6
Tuna in water	*	*	4.3
Tuna Sandwich	*	*	2.1
Tuna, in oil	*	*	1.9
Turkey	*	*	2.1
Turkey Sandwich	*	*	2.1
Twix®, Caramel, M&M Mars	44	63	1.1
Vanilla wafers	77	110	1.2

*GI cannot be calculated on some foods because of insufficient carbohydrate in them.

193

GLYCEMIC INDEX (GI) AND DR.SHINTANI'S FOOD MASS INDEX (SMI)			
Food Item	**GI** **(glu)**	**GI** **(bread)**	**Mass** **Index**
VEGETABLES			
Corn	55	79	5.5
Peas	48	69	7.0
Pumpkin	75	107	16.3
VEGETABLES, ROOT			
Beets	64	91	17.8
Carrots	71	101	12.7
Parsnips	97	139	6.8
Potato			
French fries	75	107	2.5
Potato, baked	85	121	5.9
Potato, boiled, mashed	73	104	6.2
Potato, canned	61	87	9.2
Potato, instant	83	119	7.0
Potato, new	62	89	9.1
Potato, sweet	54	77	5.3
Potato, white, baked	60	86	5.9
Potato, white, boiled	56	80	6.4
Potato, white, mashed	70	100	5.2
Potato, white, steamed	65	93	6.4
Rutabaga	72	103	16.1
Taro	54	77	5.1
Yams	51	73	4.7
Vermicelli	35	50	3.0
Waffles, Aunt Jemima®	76	109	2.8
Watercress	*	*	27.3
Watermelon	72	103	17.6
Wheat cereal	41	59	9.7
Wheat cereal, quick cooking	54	77	9.1
Wheat chapatti	27	39	3.2
Wheat Crackers®, Breton	67	96	1.1

*GI cannot be calculated on some foods because of insufficient carbohydrate in them.

GLYCEMIC INDEX (GI) AND DR.SHINTANI'S FOOD MASS INDEX (SMI)			
Food Item	**GI (glu)**	**GI (bread)**	**Mass Index**
White bread	70	100	2.1
Whole wheat bread	69	99	2.2
Yams	51	73	4.7
Zucchini	*	*	32.1

*GI cannot be calculated on some foods because of insufficient carbohydrate in them.